Foreword

It is my pleasure to introduce *The ESC Handbook of Preventive Cardiology*. It is timed to complement both the current Joint European Guidelines on cardiovascular disease prevention and *The ESC Textbook of Preventive Cardiology* (2015).

While the evidence base for the prevention of cardiovascular disease (CVD) is compelling, it poses huge challenges for healthcare workers who are busy, may feel that they lack appropriate skills and training, or find textbooks and guidelines too long and complicated, and are often paid to treat sick people but not to keep people healthy.

Neither a textbook nor guidelines on CVD prevention will be effective unless the healthcare worker at the coalface feels both responsible for prevention and has the tools and skills to deliver it. *The ESC Handbook of Preventive Cardiology* has therefore been produced to assist in this process in a practical and accessible way. The emphasis is on checklists—standard operating procedures if you will—and diagrams without rehearsing the evidence base that underpins the source guidelines and textbook. It will join the ESC's European Association of Cardiovascular Prevention and Rehabilitation (EACPR) prevention toolkit that is available through the EACPR website.

I warmly welcome the Handbook and believe that it will contribute in a real and practical way to the prevention of CVD. But this is an evolving process. We are all students. The editors will welcome suggestions for the future through c.jennings@imperial.ac.uk or ian@grahams.net.

Joep Perk MD, FESC
Chair, 2012 European Guidelines on Cardiovascular
Disease Prevention in Clinical Practice and of its
Prevention Implementation Committee

The ESC Handbook of Preventive Cardiology

Putting Prevention into Practice

Edited by

Catriona Jennings

Cardiovascular Specialist Research Nurse
National Heart and Lung Institute
Imperial College London
London, UK

Ian Graham

Professor of Cardiovascular Medicine
Trinity College
Dublin, Ireland

Stephan Gielen

Deputy Director, Department of Internal Medicine,
University Hospital Halle/Saale,
Martin-Luther-University Halle-Wittenburg, Germany

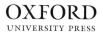

OXFORD
UNIVERSITY PRESS

EACPR
A Registered Branch of the ESC

EUROPEAN
SOCIETY OF
CARDIOLOGY®

OXFORD
UNIVERSITY PRESS

Great Clarendon Street, Oxford, OX2 6DP,
United Kingdom

Oxford University Press is a department of the University of Oxford.
It furthers the University's objective of excellence in research, scholarship,
and education by publishing worldwide. Oxford is a registered trade mark of
Oxford University Press in the UK and in certain other countries

© European Society of Cardiology 2016

The moral rights of the authors have been asserted

First Edition published in 2016

Impression: 1

Published in the United States of America by Oxford University Press
198 Madison Avenue, New York, N`Y 10016, United States of America

British Library Cataloguing in Publication Data

Data available

Library of Congress Control Number: 2015958820

ISBN 978–0–19–967403–9

Printed in Great Britain by
Clays Ltd, St Ives plc

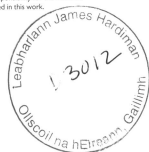

Preface

Welcome! This manual is aimed at healthcare workers who wish to improve their skills with regards to cardiovascular disease (CVD) prevention.

Atherosclerotic CVD is the biggest worldwide cause of death. Death rates are falling in Western Europe but are more variable in the East. They are rising rapidly in the developing world including China and India. Despite improvements in lipid levels and smoking in the West, overweight and consequent diabetes are increasing in most countries worldwide.

CVD relates primarily to modifiable lifestyle factors and is therefore substantially preventable.

As you will see from the resources outlined at the end of this preface, there are a plethora of textbooks and guidelines relating to the prevention of CVD. Why then yet another work on prevention? Guidelines are a waste of time unless implemented. Our aim is to produce a 'how-to' manual to assist the busy healthcare professional to achieve best practice with regard to optimal CVD prevention. This is not another textbook but rather a compendium of standard operating procedures or checklists, backed up by figures and not overburdened with pages of text.

We focus on the needs of the individual healthcare worker, while acknowledging that such efforts must be complemented by multidisciplinary, societal, and community-based strategies. Virtually everything that is in this manual can be referenced to the above resources. European Society of Cardiology (ESC) Guidelines insist on evidence grading. Grading is fine if undertaken methodically (and not just putting a number on the author's opinion). We have taken careful note of the gradings but will not transcribe them in this text although comments are occasionally in order. Reliance on randomised control trials, while generally appropriate, poses a problem in that it will tend to favour drug treatments over lifestyle measures.

So, how can you make a start to improving your preventive practice?

1. Get a feel for this book and its layout by flicking through the pages.
2. Familiarize yourself with the range of resources listed in the next section.
3. Skim read them initially so as not to get bogged down.
4. If you only have time to use one paper resource, make it the pocket guidelines, or even the one-page aide-memoire, the 'European SCORE Memocard' available for download from the Prevention Toolkit website listed in 'Resources'. But try to find time to play with HeartScore and perhaps the Guideline Learning Tool.
5. Every patient contact is an opportunity to ask: 'Is this person at risk? Can I measure it and initiate help right now?'

6. Don't forget one of the biggest failings in prevention—to check the risk of relatives of high-risk subjects.

7. Understand some of the factors that impede effective prevention and think: which are manageable? (See chapters in Part 2.)

8. Consider if you have the resources to plan to audit your efforts (see Chapter 22)—this helps to plan more effective practice and is increasingly required by training and regulatory authorities anyway.

9. You may not have the time, training or resources to do everything. A key point is to be your patient's ally and to discuss one change that they may succeed with before fixing everything.

10. If the advice in this handbook is too detailed, focus on the key messages.

Resources

Major resources are now available to help the healthcare professional with regards to the prevention of CVD. These include the ESC Joint European Guidelines on CVD prevention in clinical practice (2012 and 2016), and *The ESC Textbook of Preventive Cardiology* (2015).

The Joint Guidelines are complemented by more specialist guidelines from some of the participating bodies:

- ESC and European Atherosclerosis Society on dyslipidaemias (2011 and 2016)
- ESC and European Society for Hypertension on hypertension (2013)
- ESC and European Association for the Study of Diabetes on diabetes, pre-diabetes, and cardiovascular disease (2013).

These and more guidelines are readily available by entering 'ESC' into your search engine, or directly through http://www.escardio.org/guidelines. In the 'Guidelines' section of the website you will also find take-home messages and a prevention slide kit.

Additional material is available through the European Association of Cardiovascular Disease Prevention and Rehabilitation (EACPR) website. Enter 'EACPR' into your search engine, or go directly to http://www.escardio.org/communities/EACPR.

Click on the button labelled 'Prevention Toolbox' for direct access to:

- Links to the guidelines
- SCORE (high and low-risk) posters for estimation of 10-year risk
- Link to HeartScore, the ESC's interactive risk estimation and management tool, based on SCORE. HeartScore includes a number of country-specific versions and other countries are advised when to use the high- or low-risk versions as appropriate
- The Guideline Learning Tool, a highly interactive, case-based learning guide to the Joint Guidelines
- A prevention e-toolkit which can be downloaded. This includes a single-page summary card.

Pocket versions of the Guidelines and a Prevention Toolkit are distributed at the Congresses of the ESC and EACPR.

Well done! You're well on the way already.

Contents

Abbreviations

ACC	American College of Cardiology
ACEI	angiotensin-converting enzyme inhibitor
AHA	American Heart Association
ARB	angiotensin receptor blocker
BACPR	British Association for Cardiovascular Prevention and Rehabilitation
BIA	bioelectrical impedance analysis
BMI	body mass index
BP	blood pressure
CAD	coronary artery disease
CHD	coronary heart disease
CIMT	carotid intima–media thickness
CK	creatine kinase
CMR	cardiac magnetic resonance
CRP	C-reactive protein
CT	computed tomography
CVD	cardiovascular disease
CYP	cytochrome P450
ECG	electrocardiogram
ED	erectile dysfunction
ESH	European Society of Hypertension
GFR	glomerular filtration rate
GI	glycaemic index
GP	general practitioner
HADS	Hospital Anxiety and Depression Scale
HDL	high-density lipoprotein
hsCRP	high-sensitivity C-reactive protein
INR	international normalized ratio
ISH	International Society of Hypertension
LDL	low-density lipoprotein
MET	metabolic equivalent of task
MI	myocardial infarction
MPI	myocardial perfusion imaging

MUFA	monounsaturated fatty acid
NRT	nicotine replacement therapy
PROM	patient-reported outcome measure
PUFA	polyunsaturated fatty acid
RCT	randomized controlled trial
SBP	systolic blood pressure
SCORE	systematic coronary risk estimation
SFA	saturated fatty acid
SSRI	serotonin reuptake inhibitor
TC	total cholesterol
TCA	tricyclic antidepressant
TFA	trans fatty acid
UKPDS	United Kingdom Prospective Diabetes Study
ULN	upper limit of normal
US	ultrasound scan
WC	waist circumference
WHO	World Health Organization
WHR	waist:hip ratio

Contributors

Christian Albus

Department of Psychosomatics and Psychotherapy, University of Cologne, Cologne, Germany

Felicity Astin

Calderdale and Huddersfield NHS Trust and University of Huddersfield, Huddersfield, West Yorkshire, UK

Alison Atrey

Imperial College London, UK

Pascale Benlian

University of Lille, Lille, France

Henry Boardman

Department of Cardiovascular Medicine, John Radcliffe Hospital, Oxford, UK

Renata Cifkova

Center for Cardiovascular Prevention, Thomayer University Hospital, Prague, Czech Republic

Susan Connolly

National Heart and Lung Institute, Imperial College London, London, UK

Marie-Therese Cooney

St. Vincent's Hospital, Elm Park, Dublin, Ireland

Guy De Backer

Division of Cardiology, University of Ghent, Ghent, Belgium

Kate Exley

University of Leeds, UK

Miles Fisher

Glasgow Royal Infirmary, Glasgow, UK

Irene Gibson

West of Ireland Cardiac Foundation, Croi Heart and Stroke Centre, Galway, Ireland

Ian Graham

Trinity College, Dublin, Ireland

Graham Jackson

London Bridge Hospital, London, UK

Rod Jackson

School of Population Health, Auckland, New Zealand

Catriona Jennings

Department of Cardiovascular Medicine, Imperial College London, London, UK

Kornelia Kotseva

Imperial College London, London, UK

Paul Leeson

Department of Cardiovascular Medicine, John Radcliffe Hospital, Oxford, UK

Alessandro Mezzani

Cardiac Rehabilitation Division, Salvatore Maugeri Foundation, IRCCS, Scientific Institute of Veruno, Veruno, Italy

Massimo Piepoli

Heart Failure Unit, G Da Saliceto Hospital, Piacenza, Italy

Andrew Pipe

Division of Prevention and
Rehabilitation, University of Ottawa,
Ottawa, Canada

Zeljko Reiner

University Hospital Center Zagreb,
University of Zagreb, Zagreb, Croatia

Serena Tonstad

The School of Public Health, Loma
Linda University, Loma Linda, CA, USA;
Department of Endocrinology, Morbid
Obesity and Preventive Medicine,
Section for Preventive Cardiology, Oslo
University Hospital, Oslo, Norway

Kathy Whyte

Kathywhytehealth: http://www.
kathywhytehealth.ie/

Part 1

What is prevention and why do we need it?

Chapter 1

Why do we need cardiovascular disease prevention?

Introduction to cardiovascular disease

Medicine is full of waffle. Here are the ten points to make you a prevention guru:

1. Cardiovascular disease (CVD) is the major cause of death in Europe and most of the rest of the world and a major drain on health resources.

2. The underlying atherosclerosis develops very slowly, starting in childhood or even *in utero*, but is often advanced and hard to reverse by the time that symptoms occur.

3. Many deaths occur rapidly, before medical help is available. This is because they are caused by abrupt rupture of an atherosclerotic plaque, for example, in a coronary artery. Therefore treatments are often *palliative* (advanced disease) or *inapplicable* (person is dead before help arrives).

4. There has been a gradual recognition that CVD relates to modifiable risk factors. Over 60 years of methodical research has separated incidental associations from actual causes. Cigarettes smoking, a high-fat diet with consequent hyperlipidaemia, and hypertension are all *causes*. Hundreds of other risk factors have been identified but are relatively minor players compared with the 'big three'.

5. Risk factors tend to cluster together with additive or multiplicative effects. This is the basis of the total risk approach to CVD prevention: see one, look for others, and estimate total risk. Central obesity tends to drive diabetes, hypertension, and dyslipidaemias.

6. There is now unequivocal evidence that prevention through risk factor management reduces mortality and morbidity. The evidence base that effective management of hypertension and hyperlipidaemia reduces both mortality and morbidity is as strong as for any intervention in the history of medicine. While not amenable to randomized control trials, observational studies indicate that the effects of smoking cessation are even stronger.

7. A family history of premature CVD occasionally flags a genetic cause such as familial hyperlipidaemia, but more often it signals a shared high-risk lifestyle. Check all family members!

8. It's not just a cliché—the poor really do die young. Social deprivation is a powerful 'cause of the causes' of CVD. It probably underpins the rise in CVD in Eastern Europe, and there is often an inverse relationship between need and resources.

9. Population versus high-risk approach: the great Geoffrey Rose taught us that most deaths come from people at only modestly increased risk, simply because they are vastly more numerous than very high-risk people (see point 8). But as *individuals*, high-risk people gain most by risk factor change. So, your efforts to find and help such people must be complemented by an integrated community approach. (Don't forget that you are the expert and entitled to lobby for both approaches.)

10. Risk factor management has major added value in also helping to prevent other chronic diseases such as chronic lung disease, diabetes, and certain cancers.

Chapter 2

What is a high-risk patient?

Key messages

- Understand that, in most people, CVD risk results from the combined effect of several risk factors.
- Similarly, that maximum benefit arises from attending to all risk factors.
- That the higher the risk of an individual, the greater the benefit of managing risk.
- Be conversant with the categories of risk outlined in Table 2.1 because these determine the intensity of intervention.

Summary

- In apparently healthy people, CVD risk is usually the product of several risk factors. At any given cholesterol or blood pressure (BP) level, risk may vary tenfold depending on the presence of other risk factors. Risk is even higher in those with established disease. Current European guidelines define four categories of risk based on these principles (see Table 2.1). Those at highest risk gain most from risk factor management.
- This pattern of a strong direct association between the magnitude of a person's pre-intervention total CVD risk and the magnitude of treatment benefits appears to apply to most CVD risk prevention interventions. Therefore, the choice and intensity of preventive interventions should be informed primarily by a person's total CVD risk rather than by levels of individual risk factors.

The association between total CVD risk and the benefits of prevention

- The magnitude of cardiovascular benefits from preventive interventions is determined mainly by a person's *total CVD risk*, rather than by the level of an individual risk factor or how much a risk factor is lowered. This is demonstrated in Fig. 2.1, a meta-analysis of trials of low-density lipoprotein cholesterol (LDL-C) lowering.

Table 2.1 Priorities for CVD prevention

Very high risk	Subjects with any of the following: Documented CVD Type 2 diabetes, or type 1 diabetes with one or more cardiovascular risk factors and/or target organ damage (such as microalbuminuria) Severe chronic kidney disease (eGFR <30 mL/min/1.73 m²) SCORE ≥10%
High risk	Markedly elevated single risk factors such as: Familial dyslipidaemias Severe hypertension Diabetes mellitus (type 1 or type 2) but without CV risk factors or target organ damage Moderate chronic kidney disease (eGFR 30–59 mL/min/1.73 m²) SCORE ≥5% and <10%
Moderate risk	SCORE ≥1% and <5%, further modulated by:
	Family history of premature CAD / Abdominal obesity / Low physical activity levels / Low HDL-C / Elevated triglycerides / Elevated hsCRP / Social class
Low risk	SCORE <1% and free of qualifiers

CAD, coronary artery disease; GFR, glomerular filtration rate; HDL-C, high-density lipoprotein cholesterol; hsCRP, high-sensitivity C-reactive protein; SCORE, Systematic COronary Risk Estimation.

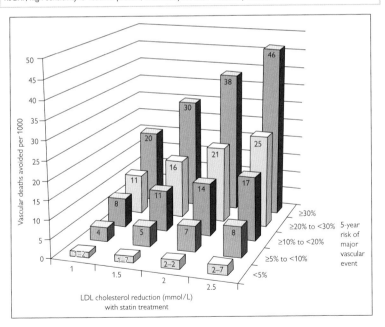

Figure 2.1 Vascular deaths avoided through lowering LDL-C with statins by different amounts in people at different levels of pre-intervention *total CVD risk* (based on a meta-analysis of randomized controlled trials (RCTs) of statins).

Reprinted from *Lancet*, 280/9841, Cholesterol Treatment Trialists' (CTT) Collaborators, The effects of lowering LDL cholesterol with statin therapy in people at low risk of vascular disease: meta-analysis of individual data from 27 randomised trials, 581–90, Copyright (2012) with permission from Elsevier.

- A similar meta-analysis has shown that the benefits of lowering BP are also determined primarily by a person's total CVD risk rather than by the BP level or by how much BP is lowered.

Rl
Estimating total CVD risk

- *Total CVD risk* (i.e. the probability of having a CVD event during a defined time period) is determined by the combined effect of all CVD risk factors present.
- People with identical BP levels (or another single risk factor) may have more than tenfold differences in their *total CVD risk*, depending on the presence or absence of other CVD risk factors, as illustrated in Fig. 2.2.
- CVD risk factors interact, sometime multiplicatively, so it is not possible to estimate a person's *total CVD risk* simply by summing risk factors.
- *Total CVD risk* is typically estimated using a two-step process. First, people with evidence of pre-existing CVD or end-organ damage are classified at very high risk. For the remainder, *total CVD risk* is usually estimated using a chart or computer program derived from mathematical risk algorithms that are based on studies that have followed people after measuring their CVD risk factor profiles.
- A wide range of risk charts and computer algorithms are available for estimating total CVD risk (e.g. Systematic COronary Risk Estimation (SCORE)).

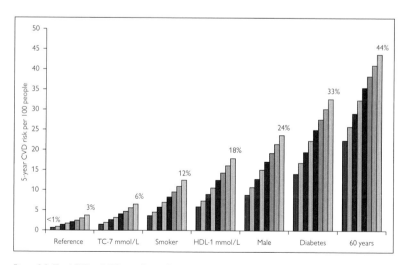

Figure 2.2 Total CVD risk (%) over 5 years by systolic BP (SBP) level (each set of vertical bars represents the same range of SBP levels from 110 to 180 mmHg) depending on the accumulation of other CVD risk factors. Reference category are 50-year-old, non-smoking, non-diabetic women with total cholesterol (TC) = 4.0 mmol/L and HDL = 1.6 mmol/L.

Reprinted from *Lancet*, 365, Jackson R, Lawes C, Bennett D, Milne R, Rodgers A., Treatment with drugs to lower blood pressure and blood cholesterol based on an individual's absolute cardiovascular risk, 434–41, Copyright (2005) with permission from Elsevier.

Categories of total CVD risk

- The European Joint Societies Task Force on Cardiovascular Disease Prevention in Clinical Practice state that 'the higher the risk the greater the benefits from preventive efforts'.
- The Task Force uses four priority groups (see Table 2.1) to classify people according to their estimated risk. Those at highest risk gain most from risk factor management.
- Each of the common risk reduction interventions (smoking cessation, lipid lowering, BP lowering, antiplatelet therapies) is estimated to reduce the total CVD risk by 15–30% over about 5 years, while a combination of at least three of these interventions is likely to reduce risk by over 50%.
- Therefore after categorizing a person according to their total CVD risk, it is possible to estimate the approximate number of people with a similar risk who would need to be treated to prevent one CVD event over a defined time period.

Key reading

Blood Pressure Lowering Treatment Trials (BPLTT) Collaboration. Blood pressure-lowering treatment based on cardiovascular risk: a meta-analysis of individual patient data. *Lancet* 2014; 384:591–98.

Cholesterol Treatment Trialists' (CTT) Collaborators. The effects of lowering LDL cholesterol with statin therapy in people at low risk of vascular disease: meta-analysis of individual data from 27 randomised trials. *Lancet* 2012; 380:581–90.

European Society for Cardiology, European Association for Cardiovascular Prevention & Rehabilitation. *HeartScore*. [Online] http://www.heartscore.org/Pages/welcome.aspx

Jackson R, Lawes C, Bennett D, *et al.* Treatment with drugs to lower blood pressure and blood cholesterol based on an individual's absolute cardiovascular risk. *Lancet* 2005; 365:434–41.

Perk J, De Backer G, Gohlke H, *et al.* European Guidelines on cardiovascular disease prevention in clinical practice (version 2012). The Fifth Joint Task Force of the European Society of Cardiology and Other Societies on Cardiovascular Disease Prevention in Clinical Practice (constituted by representatives of nine societies and by invited experts). *Eur Heart J* 2012; 33:1635–701.

Wald NJ, Law MR. A strategy to reduce cardiovascular disease by more than 80%. *BMJ* 2003; 326:1419.

Chapter 3

How to assess risk

Key messages

- Understand the rationale for total risk estimation outlined in Chapter 2.
- Consider risk assessment at every person/patient contact, especially if one or more risk factors are present or if there is a strong family history of CVD.
- Be familiar with the guideline categories of CVD risk because these determine priorities.
- Know that CVD often results from several risk factors and when and how to use a risk assessment tool such as SCORE.
- SCORE is used in apparently healthy people. Those with established CVD are automatically at high risk for further events.
- Understand that highest-risk individuals gain most from risk factor management.
- Understand the concepts of relative risk and risk age when counselling young people.
- Develop an agreed management and follow-up plan (see chapters in Part 2).

Summary

- High-risk and population approaches to CVD prevention are complementary, not competitive.
- High-risk individuals gain most from risk factor control.
- People with several risk factors may be at higher risk than someone with a single more dramatic risk factor—hence the principle of total risk estimation.
- SCORE is the recommended European risk estimation system. There are versions for high- and low-risk countries.
- A young person's absolute risk may be misleadingly low.
- As many women as men die from CVD; they just do it later.

Introduction

The high-risk approach to prevention of CVD is based on identifying those at highest cardiovascular risk and directing the most intensive risk factor management towards

Gender	Age (years)	Cholesterol (mmol/L)	Systolic blood pressure (mmHg)	Smoker	SCORE risk
Woman	60	8	120	No	2
Woman	60	7	140	No	5
Man	60	6	160	Yes	8
Man	60	5	180	Yes	21

Table 3.1 SCORE estimates of 10-year risk of fatal CVD in people with different risk factor combinations

those at highest risk because they will gain most from risk factor management. That said, the high-risk strategy must be complemented by a population strategy which aims at reducing risk factor levels in the entire population, generally by encouraging a healthy lifestyle, as discussed in Chapter 8. The priorities for CVD prevention are outlined in Table 2.1 in Chapter 2.

As shown in Table 2.1, some individuals have already declared themselves to be at increased risk, for example, those with established CVD, diabetes, or renal disease. In apparently healthy individuals, a system for estimating the risk due to the combination of their risk factors is required. This is because cardiovascular risk usually reflects the combined effects of several risk factors that may interact, sometimes multiplicatively.

'Total risk' implies an estimate of risk made by considering the effect of the major factors: age, gender, smoking, BP, and lipid levels. The term has become widely used; however, 'total risk' is not comprehensive because the effects of other risk factors are not considered except as qualifying statements.

The importance of total risk estimation before management decisions are made is illustrated in Table 2.1 in Chapter 2. Table 3.1 shows that a person with a cholesterol concentration of 8 mmol/L can be at ten times *lower* risk than someone with a cholesterol concentration of 5 mmol/L if the latter is a male hypertensive smoker.

Risk estimation systems

There are several systems available to assess total cardiovascular risk. These include the Framingham Risk Score, SCORE, ASSIGN, QRISK, Prospective Cardiovascular Münster (PROCAM), World Health Organization/International Society of Hypertension (WHO/ISH) model, the Reynolds score, Q-risk, and the 2013 American Heart Association (AHA)/American College of Cardiology (ACC) system. These have been comprehensively reviewed. SCORE is the risk estimation recommended by the European guidelines on CVD prevention and by the European guidelines on management of dyslipidaemia. HeartScore, the interactive electronic version of SCORE, is available online as part of the European Society of Cardiology (ESC) website (http://www.HeartScore.org).

SCORE

The SCORE risk function was derived from data from 11 European cohort studies. It estimates the 10-year risk of a first fatal atherosclerotic event, whether heart attack, stroke, aneurysm of the aorta, or other. Some other systems estimate coronary heart disease (CHD) risk only.

Risk of fatal CVD can be converted to risk of total (fatal + non-fatal CVD) by multiplying by three, or a little less in older people in whom a first event is more likely to be fatal.

Risk will be overestimated in populations in whom CVD is declining, and underestimated in populations in which it is decreasing. This can be dealt with by recalibration. Recalibration, using up-to-date local mortality and risk factor prevalence data, can improve the performance of risk estimation systems when applied to different populations. Examples of recalibrated SCORE charts can be viewed at http://www.heartscore.org.

The SCORE risk charts are shown in Figs 3.1–3.3, including a chart of relative risks. Instructions on their use and qualifiers follow.

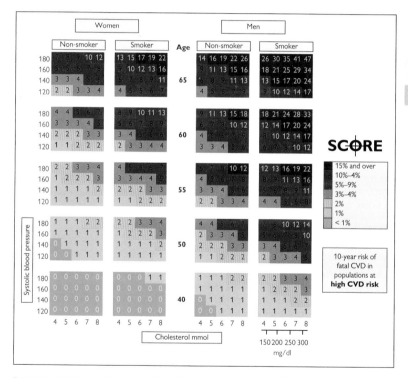

Figure 3.1 SCORE chart: 10-year risk of fatal CVD in populations at high CVD risk based on the following risk factors: age, sex, smoking, SBP, and total cholesterol (TC). Note that the risk of total (fatal + non-fatal) CVD events will be approximately three times higher than the figures given.

Reproduced from The ESC Textbook of Preventive Cardiology, Gielen et al. with permission of Oxford University Press.

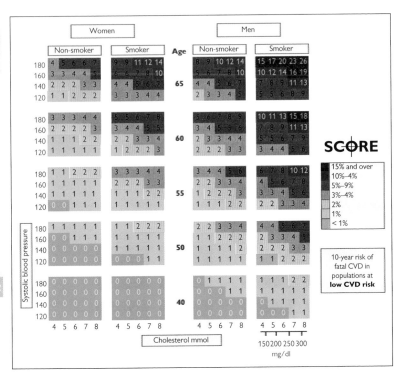

Figure 3.2 SCORE chart: 10-year risk of fatal CVD in populations at low CVD risk based on the following risk factors: age, sex, smoking, SBP, and TC.

Reproduced from *The ESC Textbook of Preventive Cardiology*, Gielen *et al.* with permission of Oxford University Press.

How to use the SCORE charts

• Use the appropriate version of the chart: the recalibrated chart if available, otherwise, the low-risk chart for the regions listed in Table 3.2, and the high-risk chart for other European countries. Of these, some are at very high risk (see Box 3.1). The charts will underestimate risk in these countries.

• Find the cell nearest to the person's age, cholesterol, and BP values, bearing in mind that risk will be higher as the person approaches the next age, cholesterol, or BP category.

• Check the qualifiers (several factors known to modify CVD risk but which are not included in SCORE should also be taken into consideration, see Box 3.1).

• Establish the total 10-year risk for fatal CVD.

Table 3.2 Regions where the low-risk version of SCORE should be used, where recalibrated versions of SCORE are available, and very high-risk regions

Low-risk regions		Recalibrated	Very high-risk regions
Andorra	Malta	Czech Republic	Armenia
Austria	Monaco	Germany	Azerbaijan
Belgium	Netherlands	Greece	Belarus
Cyprus	Norway	Netherlands	Bulgaria
Denmark	Portugal	Poland	Georgia
Finland	San Marino	Spain	Kazakhstan
France	Slovenia	Sweden	Kyrgyzstan
Germany	Spain	Slovakia	Latvia
Greece	Sweden		Lithuania
Iceland	Switzerland		Macedonia FYR
Ireland	United Kingdom		Moldova
Israel			Russia
Italy			Ukraine
Luxembourg			Uzbekistan

Communicating about CVD risk to younger people

Young people may have a low absolute risk even if they have multiple risk factors, but it will increase rapidly as they age. *Relative risk* and *cardiovascular risk age* are two ways of expressing risk which may be useful in talking with younger subjects.

Relative risk chart

Fig. 3.3 shows the relative risk which is included in the current European guidelines on CVD prevention. The numbers displayed indicate the *relative* and not the absolute risk.

Box 3.1 Qualifiers for SCORE

Risk may also be higher than indicated in the charts in:

- Sedentary individuals
- Central obesity
- Socially deprived individuals
- Ethnic minority groups
- Preclinical atherosclerosis (e.g. carotid plaque)
- Diabetes and pre-diabetes

- Low HDL-C
- Increased triglycerides (TGs)
- Increased fibrinogen
- Increased apolipoprotein B
- Increased lipoprotein (a), especially in combination with familial
- hypercholesterolaemia.

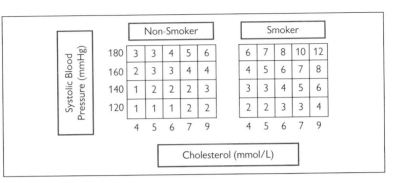

Figure 3.3 Relative risk chart.
Reproduced from *The ESC Textbook of Preventive Cardiology*, Gielen *et al.* with permission of Oxford University Press.

Thus a person in the top right-hand box has a risk that is 12 times higher than a person in the bottom left. This may be helpful when advising a young person with a *low absolute* but *high relative risk* of the need for lifestyle change.

Cardiovascular risk age

The risk age of a person with several cardiovascular risk factors is the age of a person with the same level of risk but with ideal levels of risk factors. Thus a high-risk 40-year-old may have a risk age of 60 years or more. Risk age is an intuitive and easily understood way of illustrating the likely reduction in life expectancy that a young person with a low absolute but high relative risk of CVD will be exposed to if preventive measures are not adopted.

Risk age can be estimated visually by looking at the SCORE chart (as illustrated in Fig. 3.4). Risk age is also automatically calculated as part of the latest revision of HeartScore and a table of risk ages is provided in the guidelines.

Risk age has been shown to be independent of the cardiovascular end point used, which bypasses the dilemma of whether to use a risk estimation system based on CVD mortality or on the more attractive but less reliable end point of total CVD events. Additionally, risk age can be used in any population regardless of baseline risk and of secular changes in mortality and therefore avoids the need for recalibration.

Conclusions

Estimation of total risk, using SCORE, remains a crucial part of all current guidelines. Information on relative as well as absolute risk is added to facilitate the counselling of younger people whose low absolute risk may conceal a substantial and modifiable age-related risk.

The principles of risk estimation and the definition of priorities reflect an attempt to make complex issues simple and accessible. Their very simplicity makes them vulnerable to criticism. Above all they must be interpreted in the light of both the physician's detailed knowledge of their patient and local guidance and conditions.

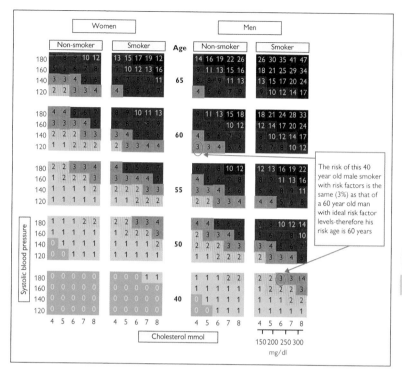

Figure 3.4 SCORE chart (for use in high-risk European regions) illustrating how the approximate risk age can be read off the chart.

Key reading

Aspelund T, Thorgeirsson G, Sigurdsson G, *et al.* Estimation of 10-year risk of fatal cardiovascular disease and coronary heart disease in Iceland with results comparable with those of the Systematic Coronary Risk Evaluation project. *Eur J Cardiovasc Prev Rehabil* 2007; 14:761–8.

Assmann G, Cullen P, Schulte H. Simple scoring scheme for calculating the risk of acute coronary events based on the 10-year follow-up of the prospective cardiovascular Munster (PROCAM) study. *Circulation* 2002; 105:310–15.

Conroy RM, Pyorala K, Fitzgerald AP, *et al.* Estimation of ten-year risk of fatal cardiovascular disease in Europe: the SCORE project. *Eur Heart J* 2003; 24:987–1003.

Cooney MT, Dudina A, D'Agostino R, *et al.* Cardiovascular risk-estimation systems in primary prevention: do they differ? Do they make a difference? Can we see the future? *Circulation* 2010; 122:300–10.

Cooney MT, Dudina AL, Graham IM. Value and limitations of existing scores for the assessment of cardiovascular risk: a review for clinicians. *J Am Coll Cardiol* 2009; 54:1209–27.

Cooney MT, Vartiainen E, Laatikainen T, et al. Cardiovascular risk age: concepts and practicalities. *Heart* 2012; 98:941–6.

Cuende JI, Cuende N, Calaveras-Lagartos J. How to calculate vascular age with the SCORE project scales: a new method of cardiovascular risk evaluation. *Eur Heart J* 2010; 31:2351–8.

D'Agostino RS, Vasan RS, Pencina MJ, et al. General cardiovascular risk profile for use in primary care: the Framingham Heart Study. *Circulation* 2008; 117:743–53.

De Backer G, Ambrosioni E, Borch-Johnsen K, et al. European guidelines on cardiovascular disease prevention in clinical practice: third joint task force of European and other societies on cardiovascular disease prevention in clinical practice (constituted by representatives of eight societies and by invited experts). *Eur J Cardiovasc Prev Rehabil* 2003; 10(4):S1–S10.

Graham I, Atar D, Borch-Johnsen K, et al. European guidelines on cardiovascular disease prevention in clinical practice: full text. Fourth Joint Task Force of the European Society of Cardiology and other societies on cardiovascular disease prevention in clinical practice (constituted by representatives of nine societies and by invited experts). *Eur J Cardiovasc Prev Rehabil* 2007; 14 Suppl 2:S1–113.

Hippisley-Cox J, Coupland C, Vinogradova Y, et al. Derivation and validation of QRISK, a new cardiovascular disease risk score for the United Kingdom: prospective open cohort study. *BMJ* 2007; 335:136.

Perk J, De Backer G, Gohlke H, et al. European Guidelines on cardiovascular disease prevention in clinical practice (version 2012): The Fifth Joint Task Force of the European Society of Cardiology and Other Societies on Cardiovascular Disease Prevention in Clinical Practice (constituted by representatives of nine societies and by invited experts). *Eur Heart J* 2012; 33(13):1635–701.

Reiner Z, Catapano AL, De Backer G, et al. ESC/EAS Guidelines for the management of dyslipidaemias: the Task Force for the management of dyslipidaemias of the European Society of Cardiology (ESC) and the European Atherosclerosis Society (EAS). *Eur Heart J* 2011; 32:1769–818.

Ridker PM, Buring JE, Rifai N, et al. Development and validation of improved algorithms for the assessment of global cardiovascular risk in women: the Reynolds Risk Score. *JAMA* 2007; 297:611–19.

Ridker PM, Paynter NP, Rifai N, et al. C-reactive protein and parental history improve global cardiovascular risk prediction: the Reynolds Risk Score for men. *Circulation* 2008; 118:2243–51.

Rose G. Sick individuals and sick populations. *Int J Epidemiol* 1985; 14:32–8.

Woodward M, Brindle P, Tunstall-Pedoe H. Adding social deprivation and family history to cardiovascular risk assessment: the ASSIGN score from the Scottish Heart Health Extended Cohort (SHHEC). *Heart* 2007; 93:172–6.

World Health Organization. *Prevention of Cardiovascular Disease: Guidelines for Assessment and Management of Cardiovascular Risk*. Geneva: WHO; 2007.

Chapter 4

Biomarkers in risk assessment

Key messages

- Understand that novel biomarkers have only limited additional value when added to CVD risk assessment with the SCORE or other risk algorithm.
- They may help to refine risk estimation in those at intermediate risk
- They may also signal a need to try harder with conventional risk factors.
- Understand also that no benefit has derived from trials of reducing these factors.

Summary

- High-sensitivity C-reactive protein (hsCRP) should not be measured in asymptomatic low-risk individuals and high-risk patients to assess 10-year risk of CVD.
- HsCRP may be measured as part of refined risk assessment in patients with an unusual or moderate CVD risk profile.
- Similar conclusions apply to fibrinogen.
- Homocysteine may be measured as part of a refined risk assessment in patients with an unusual or moderate CVD risk profile.
- Lipoprotein-associated phospholipase A_2 (Lp-PLA$_2$) may be measured as part of a refined risk assessment in patients at high risk of a recurrent acute atherothrombotic event.

Introduction

Although the number of potential risk markers increases year by year, few have proved to have significant clinical utility when exposed to evidence-based grading.

After removing biomarkers relevant to glucose and lipid metabolism, the current European guidelines on CVD prevention identify two groups of systemic biomarkers with sufficient evidence for roles in either inflammation or thrombosis and which are therefore potentially relevant to CVD risk assessment:

- Inflammatory: hsCRP and fibrinogen
- Thrombotic: homocysteine and Lp-PLA$_2$.

Inflammatory: hsCRP and fibrinogen

HsCRP has shown consistency across large prospective studies as a risk factor integrating multiple metabolic and low-grade inflammatory markers underlying the development of unstable atherosclerotic plaques, with a magnitude of effect matching that of classical major risk factors.

HsCRP has been used in individuals showing a moderate level of risk from clinical assessment of major CVD risk factors. However, several weak points argue against including this novel biomarker for risk assessment in general prevention guidelines:

- Multiplicity of confounders: dependence on other classical major risk factors
- Lack of precision: narrow diagnostic window for hsCRP level and risk of CVD
- Lack of specificity: similar level of risk for other non-cardiovascular causes of morbidity and mortality (e.g. other low-grade inflammatory diseases)
- Lack of dose–effect or causality relationship between changes in hsCRP level and risk of CVD
- Lack of specific therapeutic strategies or agents targeting circulating CRP and showing reduction in CVD incidence
- Higher cost of test compared with classical biological risk factors (e.g. blood glucose and lipids).

Fibrinogen is also related to risk and similar conclusions can be drawn. In addition, no effective management strategy is available apart from stopping smoking.

Thrombotic: homocysteine and Lp-PLA$_2$

Homocysteine

Homocysteine has shown precision as an independent risk factor for CVD. The magnitude of effect on risk is modest, and consistency is often lacking, mainly due to nutritional, metabolic (e.g. renal disease), and lifestyle confounders. In addition, intervention studies using B vitamins to reduce plasma homocysteine have not been shown to reduce the risk of CVD. Together with the cost of the test, homocysteine remains a 'second-line' marker for CVD risk estimation.

Lp-PLA$_2$

Lp-PLA$_2$ has recently emerged as a marker with high consistency and precision as an independent risk factor for plaque rupture and atherothrombotic events. The magnitude of effect on risk remains modest at the level of the general population; study limitations or bias is present. Together with the cost of the test, Lp-PLA$_2$ remains a 'second-line' marker for CVD risk estimation.

Most important new information

Overall, emerging validated biomarkers may add value in a context of specialized practice, to more precisely assess CVD risk in specific subgroups of patients at intermediate, unusual, or undefined levels of risk (e.g. asymptomatic patients without multiple major classical risk factors, but affected with a rare metabolic, inflammatory, endocrine, or social condition associated with atherosclerosis or displaying signs of atherosclerosis progression).

Overall, emerging validated biomarkers may add value in a context of specialized practice, to more precisely assess CVD risk in specific subgroups of patients at intermediate, unusual, or undefined levels of risk such as asymptomatic patients without multiple major classical risk factors and those affected with a rare metabolic, inflammatory, or endocrine condition associated with atherosclerosis or displaying signs of aggressive progression of atherosclerosis.

Key reading

Berger JS, Jordan CO, Lloyd-Jones D, et al. Screening for cardiovascular risk in asymptomatic patients. *J Am Coll Cardiol* 2010; 55:1169–77.

Clarke R, Halsey J, Lewington S, et al. Effects of lowering homocysteine levels with B vitamins on cardiovascular disease, cancer, and cause-specific mortality: meta-analysis of 8 randomized trials involving 37 485 individuals. *Arch Intern Med* 2010; 170:1622–31.

Garza CA, Montori VM, McConnell JP, et al. Association between lipoprotein-associated phospholipase A2 and cardiovascular disease: a systematic review. *Mayo Clin Proc* 2007; 82:159–65.

Kaptoge S, Di Angelantonio E, Lowe G, et al. C-reactive protein concentration and risk of coronary heart disease, stroke, and mortality: an individual participant meta-analysis. *Lancet* 2010; 375:132–40.

Kaptoge S, White IR, Thompson SG, et al. Associations of plasma fibrinogen levels with established cardiovascular disease risk factors, inflammatory markers, and other characteristics: individual participant meta-analysis of 154,211 adults in 31 prospective studies: the fibrinogen studies collaboration. *Am J Epidemiol* 2007; 166:867–79.

Perk J, De Backer G, Gohlke H, et al. European Guidelines on cardiovascular disease prevention in clinical practice (version 2012). The Fifth Joint Task Force of the European Society of Cardiology and Other Societies on Cardiovascular Disease Prevention in Clinical Practice (constituted by representatives of nine societies and by invited experts). *Eur Heart J* 2012; 33:1635–701.

Chapter 5

Imaging in risk assessment

Key messages

- Understand the imaging modalities available.
- Know that, in apparently health people, the main role of imaging is in refining risk estimation in those at intermediate risk.

Summary

- Imaging includes computed tomography (CT), cardiac magnetic resonance (CMR), ultrasound examination of arteries and the heart, myocardial perfusion imaging (MPI), and coronary arteriography.
- Many of these modalities are expensive and some involve exposure to radiation.
- They are capable of refining risk estimation in apparently healthy people at intermediate risk.
- They have a more major role to play in the assessment of those with established CVD, but this is more in the realm of clinical management and beyond the scope of this manual.

Introduction

Imaging plays an increasing role in preventive medicine, particularly in cardiology. There are several different modalities for clinicians to choose from:

- CT: involves ionizing radiation and is used to assess coronary artery disease (CAD), either through a coronary calcium score or CT coronary angiography.
- CMR: involves non-ionizing radiation. Good for looking at cardiac structure and function and rarely limited by body habitus. Used for investigating cardiomyopathies, aortic disease, and CAD in terms of myocardial stress perfusion.
- Ultrasound scan: used to assess atherosclerosis in the form of plaques and carotid stenoses. Main measure in primary prevention is of carotid intima–media thickness (CIMT), a surrogate marker of cardiovascular morbidity and mortality. Ultrasound is non-invasive and involves no radiation. Recent evidence favours assessing both CIMT and plaque burden.
- Echocardiography: readily available and low risk. Uses ultrasound to look at cardiac structure and function and therefore good for investigation of cardiomyopathies, aortic disease, and CAD (as stress echocardiography).
- MPI: involves ionizing radiation. Injection of myocardial tracer with stress allows assessment of perfusion of different areas of the myocardium. Used to assess CAD in intermediate and high-risk populations.

- Coronary angiography: invasive procedure, involves ionizing radiation and is used to assess CAD in high-risk populations. A catheter is placed via a peripheral artery (usually radial or femoral) consecutively into the origins of the left and right coronary arteries and contrast medium ('dye') injected. Simultaneous fluoroscopy visualizes the coronary artery lumens and stenoses are identified.

Which prevention guidelines include imaging?

American College of Cardiology/American Heart Association: Guideline on the assessment of cardiovascular risk (2013).[1]

- CT calcium scoring may be considered to inform treatment decision (IIb).
- CIMT for routine risk assessment for a first atherosclerotic cardiovascular disease event is not recommended (III).

American Society of Echocardiography (ASE): Use of carotid ultrasound to identify subclinical vascular disease and evaluate cardiovascular disease risk: a consensus statement (2009).[2]

- Measuring CIMT and identification of carotid plaques (focal areas where the wall thickness is increased by at least 50% compared to the surrounding vessel wall) is most useful in individuals at intermediate risk (6–10% 10-year) and without established vascular disease where the results might alter management.

ESC et al.: European Guidelines on cardiovascular disease prevention in clinical practice (version 2012).[3]

- Measurement of CIMT and/or carotid plaques should be considered in asymptomatic adults at moderate risk (IIa B).
- CT calcium scoring should be considered in asymptomatic adults at moderate risk (IIa B).

European Society of Hypertension (ESH) and European Society of Cardiology (ESC): Guidelines for the management of arterial hypertension (2013):[4]

In individuals with hypertension:

- Echo should be considered when heart disease (such as LVH or left atrial dilatation) is suspected (IIa B).
- Ultrasound of carotid arteries should be considered particularly in the elderly (IIa B).
- Fundoscopy to examine the retina should be considered in difficult to control hypertensives (IIa C). It is not recommended in mild-moderate hypertension without DM, except in young patients (III C).
- Brain imaging (CT or MRI) should be considered for patients with cognitive decline to identify infarction, microbleeds and white matter lesions (IIb C).

Is there evidence that imaging modalities refine risk scores for cardiovascular disease?

Calcium scoring has been shown to independently predict CHD outcomes above and beyond risk scores.[5] A strategy of scanning as part of risk factor assessment demonstrated that patients who had CT calcium scoring had improved risk factor modification at 4 years, compared to those who just used a conventional risk factor analysis (EISNER study).[6]

The SHAPE guideline[7] recommends non-invasive screening of all asymptomatic men (45–75 years) and women (55–75 years), except those at low risk, to detect and treat those with subclinical atherosclerosis. This is unlikely to be economically realistic for developing countries.

Primary prevention

Patients who are asymptomatic but at intermediate/high risk

Carotid artery ultrasound

CIMT is a predictor of ischaemic coronary events and stroke (relative risk increases by ~15% for every 0.1 mm increase in CIMT). CIMT can regress with risk factor modification such as BP control and cholesterol lowering. However, serial scans have not been shown to benefit individuals. Recently some guidelines have questioned whether measurement of CIMT by itself is sufficient and suggested that identification of carotid plaques is also important. Currently, as shown in the section above, the guidelines are not consistent regarding the use of carotid ultrasound imaging in risk stratification.

Coronary calcium scoring

Coronary calcium score is based on quantification of calcium to which an Agatston score is given: 0 = very unlikely to have atherosclerosis, 1–400 = likely atherosclerosis, higher than 400 = severe atherosclerosis. Coronary calcification is a surrogate marker for atherosclerotic plaque and rarely occurs in other contexts, except renal failure. There is a good correlation between calcification and plaque burden but a weak correlation with stenosis severity on invasive angiography. In the United Kingdom, the National Institute for Health and Care Excellence (NICE) recommends it as the test of choice for those with suspected stable angina and a CAD risk score between 10% and 29%. A score higher than the median is associated with an odds ratio of 4.2 for myocardial infarction (MI) or death. However, the strength of the test lies in its good negative predictive value of 93–100%, but it has a poor positive predictive value of 50–100%. Problems with the calcium score are also that not all plaques are calcified, and the degree of calcification does not correlate with likelihood of rupture. In men under 40 years and women under 50 years there are typically very low levels of detectable calcium.

Patients who are symptomatic at intermediate/high risk

Invasive coronary angiography

This is considered the gold standard test for CAD and can proceed onto intervention if disease is found. It is generally performed in subjects with convincing evidence of angina and/or evidence of significant ischaemia on non-invasive testing.

Cardiac CT angiography

CT coronary angiography takes high resolution spatial and temporal coronary images using a timed injection of CT contrast. Cardiac CT is less invasive and quicker than invasive angiography and has the potential benefit of imaging plaque, vessel wall, and lumen. It is also recommended for investigating anomalous coronary arteries. Its limitations are that it is less accurate in the presence of obesity, arrhythmias, highly calcified arteries, fast heart rates, stents, and coronary artery bypass grafts.

Stress echocardiography

Echocardiography is performed visualizing the left ventricle in different planes, whilst contrast is infused to highlight the endocardial border. The patient is then either exercised or

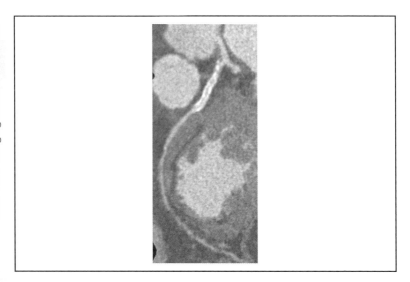

Figure 5.1 Curved multiplanar reformatted CT coronary angiogram dataset demonstrating a coronary stent in the left anterior descending artery.
Reproduced from Leeson P (ed). (2011). *Cardiovascular Imaging*, with permission from Oxford University Press.

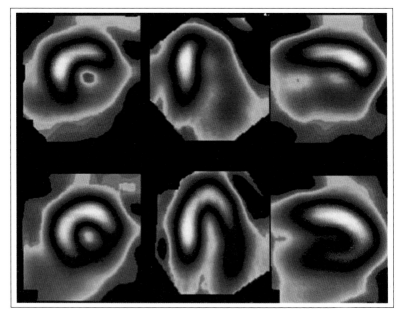

Figure 5.2 Myocardial perfusion scintigraphy planes after stress (top row) and at rest (bottom row). The images demonstrate evidence of inducible ischaemia in an inferolateral territory.
Reproduced from Leeson P (ed). (2011). *Cardiovascular Imaging*, with permission from Oxford University Press.

infused with a pharmacological inotrope or vasodilator. The resting and stress images are compared to identify functionally significant coronary artery stenoses.

Myocardial perfusion imaging

Nuclear imaging has two stages and both involve radioisotope infusion to highlight viable myocardium. A rest scan identifies baseline left ventricular function as well as viable myocardium at rest. A stress scan identifies coronary flow limitation due to a stenotic coronary artery based on identification of regions which develop relative hypoperfusion after infusion of a vasodilator.

Stress cardiac magnetic resonance

A CMR scan is performed at rest and again whilst an inotrope or vasodilator is infused. Any relative hypokinetic region at stress is likely supplied by a significantly stenotic coronary artery. If gadolinium contrast is given with the vasodilator then abnormal areas of perfusion can also be identified. Imaging the gadolinium late after the infusion can also be used to pinpoint non-viable fibrosis from previous infarcts and, vice versa, demonstrate viable myocardium which will improve with revascularization.

Secondary prevention

Post-MI risk stratification (angiography/stress imaging)

Patients post MI, whilst in-patients in most cases, should have investigations to guide potential revascularization and stratify risk. Invasive angiography to identify the culprit

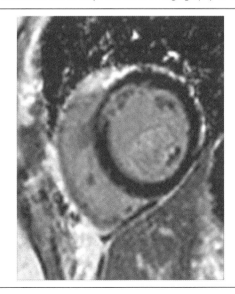

Figure 5.3 Patchy late gadolinium enhancement on cardiovascular magnetic resonance imaging in the superior part of the septum in a patient being investigated for a cardiomyopathy.
Reproduced from Leeson P (ed). (2011). *Cardiovascular Imaging*, with permission from Oxford University Press.

coronary artery stenosis, or stress imaging (stress echocardiography, MPI, stress/perfusion CMR) can detect the affected coronary territory and also assess the volume of ischaemic myocardium to guide any potential revascularization strategy.

Hypertension

Patients with hypertension should have echocardiography to assess for left ventricular hypertrophy which is associated 'independently of BP' with cardiovascular and all-cause mortality.

Examples of imaging modalities

See Figs 5.1–5.3.

Key reading

Leeson P (ed). *Cardiovascular Imaging*. Oxford: Oxford University Press, 2011.

References

1. Goff DC, Jr., Lloyd-Jones DM, Bennett G, *et al.* 2013 ACC/AHA guideline on the assessment of cardiovascular risk: a report of the American College of Cardiology/American Heart Association Task Force on Practice Guidelines. *J Am Coll Cardiol* 2014; 63(25 Pt B):2935–2959.

2. Stein JH, Korcarz CE, Post WS. Use of carotid ultrasound to identify subclinical vascular disease and evaluate cardiovascular disease risk: summary and discussion of the American Society of Echocardiography consensus statement. *Eur J Prev Cardiol* 2009; 12(1):34–8.

3. Perk J, De Backer G, Gohlke H, *et al.* European Guidelines on cardiovascular disease prevention in clinical practice (version 2012). The Fifth Joint Task Force of the European Society of Cardiology and Other Societies on Cardiovascular Disease Prevention in Clinical Practice (constituted by representatives of nine societies and by invited experts). *Eur Heart J* 2012; 33(13):1635–1701.

4. Mancia G, Fagard R, Narkiewicz K, *et al.* 2013 ESH/ESC Guidelines for the management of arterial hypertension: the Task Force for the management of arterial hypertension of the European Society of Hypertension (ESH) and of the European Society of Cardiology (ESC). *J Hypertens* 2013; 31(7):1281–1357.

5. Greenland P, Bonow RO, Brundage BH, *et al.* ACCF/AHA 2007 clinical expert consensus document on coronary artery calcium scoring by computed tomography in global cardiovascular risk assessment and in evaluation of patients with chest pain: a report of the American College of Cardiology Foundation Clinical Expert Consensus Task Force (ACCF/AHA Writing Committee to Update the 2000 Expert Consensus Document on Electron Beam Computed Tomography). *Circulation* 2007; 115(3):402–26.

6. Rozanski A, Gransar H, Shaw LJ, *et al.* Impact of coronary artery calcium scanning on coronary risk factors and downstream testing the EISNER (Early Identification of Subclinical Atherosclerosis by Noninvasive Imaging Research) prospective randomized trial. *J Am Coll Cardiol* 2011; 57:1622–32.

7. Naghavi M, Falk E, Hecht HS, *et al.* The first SHAPE (Screening for Heart Attack Prevention and Education) guideline. *Crit Pathw Cardiol* 2006; 5(4):187–90.

Chapter 6

Erectile dysfunction and cardiovascular risk

Key messages

- Erectile dysfunction (ED) may be a marker of silent CVD and should be systematically sought as part of risk assessment.
- Criteria to distinguish organic from psychogenic ED have been defined.
- Intensive risk factor advice should be offered to those with ED.

Summary

- ED may be a marker of silent CVD and is particularly strongly associated with CVD risk in younger people. Attention to CVD risk factors may improve ED.

Introduction

Both CVD and ED are common conditions which often coexist. Importantly, ED may precede CVD by 2–5 years in cardiac asymptomatic men and therefore act as an early marker for subsequent CVD. When assessing ED a precise diagnosis is necessary and other conditions need to be ruled out (e.g. premature ejaculation). Whilst most men with ED have a vascular aetiology, psychogenic ED also needs to be excluded (Table 6.1).

Erectile dysfunction predicting CVD events

There is now overwhelming evidence that organic ED predicts future CVD events and all-cause mortality including CVD mortality. Based on the available evidence, in 2005 the Princeton expert consensus concluded: 'The recognition of ED as a warning sign of silent vascular disease has led to the concept that a man with ED and no cardiac symptoms is a cardiac (or vascular) patient until proven otherwise'. The Paris consensus meeting in 2010 reinforced this conclusion by stating: 'ED is a marker for silent CAD that needs to be excluded'. In addition, ED predicts acute coronary syndrome in men with no previous cardiac history and mortality in men with and without a preceding cardiac history. Two meta-analyses have addressed the ED/CVD link (Table 6.2).

Table 6.1 Differential characteristics of psychogenic versus organic ED

Characteristic	Predominantly psychogenic ED	Predominantly organic ED
Onset	Acute	Gradual
Circumstances	Situational	Global
Course	Intermittent	Constant
Non-coital erection	Rigid	Poor
Nocturnal/early morning erections	Normal	Inconsistent
Psychosexual problems	Long history	Secondary to ED
Partner problems	At onset	Secondary to ED
Anxiety/fear	Primary	Secondary to ED

Age, erectile dysfunction, and risk

ED is a particularly strong predictor of CVD in younger and middle aged men. Focusing more intense risk screening, for example, with coronary CT angiography in men aged 30–60 years and aggressively addressing CVD risk factors has the potential to reduce long-term healthcare costs and improve outcomes.

Risk reduction benefit

• Lifestyle modification, including weight loss, exercise, and smoking cessation, together with CVD risk reduction have been shown to be effective in improving ED.
• No randomized control trials have been undertaken to establish whether risk factor intervention reduces risk in subjects with ED, but its association with CVD risk makes intensive risk factor advice logical

Table 6.2 Relative risk of increased events and mortality: ED versus no ED

Event	Meta-analysis 1(N = 92,757)	Meta-analysis 2(N = 36,744)
Pooled end points	1.44[a]	1.48[a]
CVD mortality	1.19	N/A
Myocardial infarction	1.62[a]	1.46[a]
Stroke	1.39[a]	1.35[a]
All-cause mortality	1.25[a]	1.19[a]

[a]All significant except CVD mortality.

> **Box 6.1 Extrapolation of data from ASCOT and CARDS**
>
> ### ASCOT (N = 19,000)
>
> - *Primary hypothesis 1*: a newer antihypertensive treatment regimen (calcium channel blocker ± an angiotensin-converting enzyme inhibitor (ACEI)) is more effective than an older regimen (beta blocker ± diuretic) in the primary prevention of CHD in patients with at least three pre-specified cardiovascular risk factors.
> - *Primary hypothesis 2*: lipid-lowering therapy with atorvastatin provides further benefit against CHD end points in asymptomatic, well-controlled hypertensive patients not considered dyslipidaemic (TC ≤6.5 mmol/L).
> - Five-year planned follow-up was terminated early after a median of 3.3 years in the lipid arm because of a highly significant reduction in the incidence of non-fatal MI and fatal CHD (combined primary end point) and stroke.
>
> ### CARDS (N = 2838)
>
> - CARDS was designed to evaluate statin therapy for primary prevention of CVD in patients with type 2 diabetes, without elevated LDL-C.
> - CARDS was also stopped 2 years early at 3.9 years, for similar reasons:
>   - A 37% reduction in the incidence of major cardiovascular end points, and a 48% reduction in the incidence of stroke.
>   - A reduction in the primary end point of major CVD events was apparent and statistically significant as early as 18 months after treatment initiation.

- Extrapolating data from two major cardiovascular studies, the Anglo-Scandinavian Cardiac Outcomes Trial (ASCOT) and the Collaborative Diabetes Atorvastatin Study (CARDS), may serve as a useful guide to risk reduction intervention in men with ED (see Box 6.1).
- Both studies showed that men of similar age and cardiovascular risk benefit significantly from cardiovascular risk reduction.
- Given that both trials were stopped in the 2–5-year window when it is known that the incidence of ED in hypertensives is 60% and in type 2 diabetes 70%, emphasizes the importance of CVD risk reduction in men with ED, as men with ED were almost certainly significantly represented in these two studies.

Recommendations

As ED manifests itself 2–5 years in advance of a cardiovascular event, it can serve as a marker and thus provides a window of opportunity for CVD prevention (see Fig. 6.1).

More detail on the management of ED can be found in the third Princeton Consensus guidelines.[1]

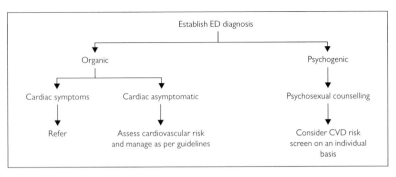

Figure 6.1 Management algorithm for erectile dysfunction.

Reference

[1]Nehra A, Jackson G, Miner M, *et al.* (2012). The Princeton III Consensus recommendations for the management of erectile dysfunction and cardiovascular disease. *Mayo Clin Proc* 87(8): 766–78.

Chapter 7

Priorities and targets

Key messages

- Become familiar with the principles of the high-risk and population approaches.
- Check your knowledge of both priorities and risk factor targets.
- Use every patient contact as an opportunity to assess risk.
- Remember to offer risk assessment to the relatives of high-risk subjects.
- For the healthcare worker, individuals at highest risk are given the highest priority for risk factor advice, and gain most from it.

Summary

- Those concerned with public health stress the need for changes at the population level because a small reduction in risk spread over the whole population confers the greatest net benefit.
- The two approaches are complementary, not competitive.
- Current European guidelines use a targeted approach, especially for blood lipids—the higher the risk, the more rigorous the target.
- Current American guidelines recommend statin treatment for all high-risk subjects (after and coupled with intensive lifestyle advice), with no cholesterol target level. This approach has had limited acceptance elsewhere.
- The European risk factor targets are summarized in this chapter and are easy to remember.

Priorities and targets

Once a child is conceived, his or her likelihood of developing a chronic disease such as CVD in later life is determined by the way of life of their parents—healthy nutrition and avoidance of alcohol and smoking in pregnancy, and a healthy parental lifestyle after delivery as the child develops.

Prevention is conventionally classified into *population* and *high-risk* approaches. This handbook is for healthcare professionals and therefore gives the highest priority to the highest-risk individuals—those with established CVD, diabetes, renal disease, and multiple risk factors. These are detailed in Chapter 2 and the global care pathway (see Fig. 19.1 in Chapter 19).

Table 7.1 Goals defined by the 2012 ESC guidelines on prevention of CVD in clinical practice	
Smoking	No exposure to tobacco in any form
Diet	Healthy diet—low in saturated fat with a focus on wholegrain products, vegetables, fruit, and fish
Physical activity	2.5 to 5 hours of moderately vigorous physical activity per week or 30–60 minutes most days
Body weight	BMI 20–25. Waist circumference <94 cm (men) or <80 cm (women)
Blood pressure	BP <140/90
Lipids	Very high risk: LDL <1.8 mmol/L or >50% reduction High risk: LDL <2.5 mmol/L Low to moderate risk: LDL <3 mmol/L HDL cholesterol: no target but >1.0 mmol/L in men and >1.2 mmol/L in women indicates lower risk Triglycerides: no target but <1.7 mmol/L indicates lower risk and higher levels indicate a need to look for other risk factors
Diabetes	HbA1C <7%, BP <140/80
Adapted from the 2012 ESC guidelines on the prevention of CVD in clinical practice.	

Having said that, most CVD deaths in fact occur in people with only modest levels of risk, *simply because there are a lot more of them*. Therefore a 'high-risk' approach alone will be comparatively ineffective and must be complemented by a population approach aimed at policies to support the avoidance of tobacco, avoidance of overweight, and encouraging and facilitating healthy eating, physical activity, and exercise.

The *priorities* for CVD prevention for individual people are summarized in Table 2.1 in Chapter 2. The risk factor *goals* are summarized in Table 7.1 and also in the global care pathway (see Fig. 19.1 in Chapter 19).

Key reading

Perk J, De Backer G, Gohlke H, et al. European Guidelines on cardiovascular disease prevention in clinical practice (version 2012). The Fifth Joint Task Force of the European Society of Cardiology and Other Societies on Cardiovascular Disease Prevention in Clinical Practice (constituted by representatives of nine societies and by invited experts). *Eur Heart J* 2012; 33:1635–701.

Part 2

Practical aspects of prevention

Chapter 8

Behavioural strategies to support and sustain lifestyle change

Key messages

- Be aware that a complex interaction exists between psychosocial factors and adverse lifestyle habits.
- Motivation and intention to initiate behaviour changes requires professional support to make a change plan which incorporates coping and enhances potential to maintain changed behaviours.
- Effective communication and counselling skills are essential to encourage initiation of behavioural changes.
- People undergoing behavioural changes require follow-up and feedback.

Summary

- This chapter focuses on psychological mechanisms relevant to behaviour change, and offers concrete information and tools to support healthy lifestyle changes.

The challenge of changing lifestyles

Relevance of psychosocial factors

Changing lifestyles is a challenge for both caregivers and patients. Whilst *healthcare policies* are very important on a population level, on an individual level, caregivers need to use established *behavioural strategies* to help their patients and families to achieve healthy lifestyle changes.

Lifestyle habits are developed during childhood and adolescence by an interaction of genetic and environmental factors, the latter comprising mainly *health behaviour modelling* from parents, peers, and the media. Subsequently, they are influenced by one's *social environment* and *socioeconomic status* as an adult. Working and living conditions frequently constitute strong barriers to lifestyle change.

The following psychosocial factors are associated with unhealthy lifestyles and can impede lifestyle change:

- Low educational level
- Low socioeconomic status

- Social isolation or low social support
- Chronic stress at work and family life
- Negative emotions like depression, anxiety, and hostility
- Cognitive impairment.

Low *socioeconomic status* and low *educational level*, for example, in manual workers or the unemployed, are associated with deprivation and poor *health literacy* (see Chapter 18), which results in unhealthy lifestyles and poor motivation for behaviour change. In addition, *financial barriers* may prevent access to health-promoting facilities and healthy food.

Feelings of *chronic stress* and negative emotions such as *depression, anxiety*, and *hostility* can be attenuated by unhealthy habits like smoking, consumption of unhealthy snacks, overeating, or excessive media consumption. Depression or anxiety often leads to poorer 'self-efficacy', which is necessary for any lifestyle change.

Social isolation and *lack of social support* are associated with chronic stress, which itself is a risk factor for unhealthy lifestyles. In addition, lack of social support (e.g. by one's spouse, close relatives, or friends) impedes behaviour change, because there is no one to encourage and help with maintenance of healthy changes.

Cognitive impairment is a major barrier to lifestyle change, because new or complex information cannot be adequately processed and translated into action. *Living alone* or *lack of social support* also increases this problem.

Whilst caregivers may not be able to influence low socioeconomic status, they can screen for psychosocial factors which may constitute important barriers to lifestyle change. Interventions can thus be tailored to individuals and provided at the appropriate intensity. Additional interventions such as stress management, psychotherapy, and antidepressant medication can also be added as appropriate.

Detailed information on how to screen and specifically manage psychosocial risk factors such as *chronic stress, depression*, and *anxiety* is given in Chapter 17. This chapter focuses on psychological mechanisms relevant to behaviour change, and offers concrete information and tools to support healthy lifestyle changes.

Psychological mechanisms relevant to behaviour change

Individuals do not simply do as they are told. Adoption of healthy lifestyles only occurs when patients are motivated. Hence, any intervention aiming at behaviour change has to start by eliciting *motivation*.

However, even in patients motivated for behaviour change, *barriers* like perceived lack of time, less knowledge, insufficient skills, or situations, where people give in to temptations, can occur ('*intention–behaviour gap*'). Thus, focusing on 'motivation' or 'intention' only, may not necessarily translate into action. In addition, although many people get engaged in healthy behaviours (e.g. after a cardiac event), *maintenance* of lifestyle change is low.

The *health action process approach* (HAPA) provides a model for predicting and modifying the adoption and maintenance of healthy behaviours (see Fig. 8.1). It identifies a distinction between motivational processes that lead to a behavioural intention (*motivational phase*), and volitional processes that lead to acting on the intention (*volitional phase*).

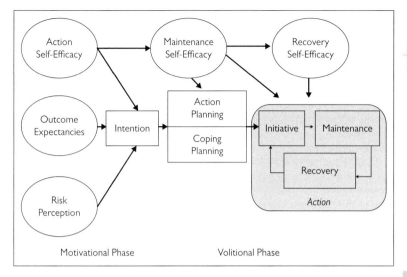

Figure 8.1 Diagram of the health action process approach.

Reproduced with permission from Schwarzer R. Modelling health behaviour change: How to predict and modify the adoption and maintenance of health behaviours. *Applied Psychology: An International Review* 2008; 57:1–29.

According to this model, interventions to support and encourage an intention to change (e.g. promotion of *risk perception, outcome expectancies*, and *action self-efficacy*), must be followed up with interventions to foster *action planning* and *coping planning* in order to initiate a repetitive, cyclic process of action, involving *initiative, maintenance*, and *recovery* after a relapse. In addition, enhancing *maintenance* and *recovery self-efficacy* is mandatory at this *volitional phase*.

So, changing behaviour is a complex process! It results in healthier lifestyle habits only in motivated individuals, who can cope with the barriers they face. In health psychology, the term 'empowerment' has been established for interventions, aiming to facilitate lifestyle change.

How to communicate effectively using cognitive behavioural strategies

Basic principles of effective communication

Adopt a *friendly* and *positive rapport* with your patients. Forcing, indoctrinating, or manipulating patients with hidden threats is counterproductive; instead, interaction with caregivers should be *attentive, empathetic*, and *facilitative*. Avoid giving complex or confusing advice.

Basic principles of effective communication[1] include the following:

- *Spend enough time* with the individual to create a therapeutic relationship—even a few more minutes can make a difference.

- *Acknowledge* the individual's personal view of his/her disease and contributing factors.

- *Encourage* expression of worries and anxieties, concerns, and self-evaluation of motivation for behaviour change and chances of success.

- *Speak to the individual in their own language* and be supportive of every improvement in lifestyle.

- *Ask questions* to check that the individual has understood the advice and has any support they require to follow it.

- *Acknowledge* that changing lifelong habits can be difficult and that a sustained gradual change is often more permanent than a rapid change.

- *Accept* that individuals may need support over a prolonged period and that repeated efforts to encourage and maintain lifestyle change may be necessary for many.

- Make sure that the information individuals are accessing is *consistent*.

The following *specific communication skills* are useful in order to establish a friendly, empathetic interaction:

- Do not blame, threaten, or be judgemental!

- Ask *open-ended questions* in order to assess true understanding, instead of a simple 'yes' or 'no' that rather could reflect social desirability.

- Use the *elicit–provide–elicit model*. Do not overwhelm your patient with facts, but ask what they want to know, then provide clear information, and then ask what he or she makes of it.

- Use *Socratic dialogue*. Don't tell your patients what to do. Rather, ask them what they feel they can do themselves to improve their health.

- Repeat, rephrase, or paraphrase important information given by the patient, in order to show that you have understood (*affirm*).

- *Roll with resistance*, that is, accept resistance as a sign of a personal dilemma. Do not argue against the patient, but show that you understand their problem, and continue to be supportive.

- Summarize important findings or decisions (*Key messages*).

Behavioural strategies to help in lifestyle change

Assess individuals' thoughts, attitudes, and beliefs concerning their willingness and per-ceived ability to change. Then, develop a *concrete lifestyle modification* plan using *shared decision-making*. Finally, provide *monitoring and feedback* in order to ensure maintenance.

'Ten strategic steps' have been recommended[1] to enhance counselling for behav-ioural change:

1. Develop a therapeutic alliance.

2. Counsel all individuals at risk of or with manifest CVD.

3. Assist individuals to understand the relationship between their behaviour and their health.

4. Explore barriers to behaviour change.
5. Establish a commitment from individuals to own their behaviour change.
6. Involve individuals in identifying and selecting the risk factors to change.
7. Use a combination of strategies including reinforcement of the individual's capacity for change.
8. Design a lifestyle-modification plan.
9. Use a multidisciplinary approach (e.g. physicians, nurses, dieticians, psychologists, etc.) whenever possible.
10. Monitor progress through follow-up contact.

Specific tools to facilitate lifestyle change

Explore beliefs, experiences, and concerns about health with your patients and share decision-making and goal setting with them and their families.

The following cognitive behavioural tools are useful:

- Motivational interviewing
- Goal setting
- Frequent monitoring and feedback.

Motivational interviewing

In order to elicit motivation for lifestyle change, use the 'Top ten useful questions' shown in Box 8.1 which can be used in a 15-minute consultation.
During the consultation, reflect on the following points:

- If the patient answers all questions positively, this demonstrates an intention to change. The next step, as explained in the HAPA model (see Fig. 8.1), is to initiate *action planning* and *coping planning*. If not, further joint negotiation on *risk perception, outcome expectancies*, and *action-self-efficacy* are required, until a firm intention has formulated (*motivational phase*).

- In this so-called *volitional phase*, there will be a potential *intention–behaviour gap*. For this reason, interventions to facilitate *action planning* should be combined with interventions to help *coping planning*, and interventions to address *action self-efficacy* should also be combined with these to address *maintenance self-efficacy*.

- For both action and coping planning, individual *goal setting* is of major importance.

Box 8.1 Top ten useful questions

- Does my patient show an appropriate risk perception (yes/no)?
- Does he tell me appropriate outcome expectancies (yes/no)?
- Are his preferences for action relevant for his health (yes/no)?
- Is he motivated for action (yes/no)?
- Does he describe enough self-efficacy to perform the desired action (yes/no)?
- Does he describe a firm intention to change (yes/no)?

Addressing self-efficacy

Global self-efficacy can be distinguished in:

- *action self-efficacy*, that is, a person has a strong, optimistic belief that his/her action will be successful with respect to the desired change
- *maintenance self-efficacy*, that is, a person is optimistic that he/she will be able to cope with barriers that may occur over time
- *recovery self-efficacy*, that is, a person is able to restore hope and find ways to restore healthy behaviour, instead of dramatizing the event due to overwhelming internal or external reasons.

Assess *action self-efficacy* with the following question: 'How confident do you feel about changing … ?'

Assess *maintenance* and *recovery self-efficacy* using the following questions:

- 'Do you think any problems will occur with your new lifestyle in the long run?'
- 'How confident do you feel about maintaining … ?'
- 'What do you think will happen if you relapse?'
- 'What kind of support would be helpful if this happens?'

Possible *barriers for maintenance* should be dealt with, for example, weight increase after smoking cessation, lack of someone to walk with in the dark, and so on. *Risk of relapse* should be anticipated, and contingency plans discussed.

Patients with psychological co-morbidities such as chronic stress, depression, and anxiety may suffer from reduced self-efficacy. In this case, additional psychosocial interventions can be valuable (see also Chapter 17).

Goal setting

Goals for behaviour change should be:

- *appropriate*, that is, address an important outcome for that individual patient
- *realistic*, that is, with high probability for successful change
- *specific*, that is, address a single, measurable outcome
- *time sensitive*, that is, a definite time point of action is defined
- *negotiated*, that is, a result of shared decision-making between caregiver and patient.

Translated into concrete recommendations, caregivers should consider the following points:

- Negotiate *every goal* with your patient, and their spouse or significant other, if applicable.
- Prioritize goals into a *hierarchical order* according to their prognostic relevance, for example, in patients with moderate obesity, stopping smoking after MI is more important than reducing weight.
- *Choose realistic goals*, for example, reducing body mass index (BMI) to recommended levels of less than 25 kg/m^2, is unrealistic for most patients. Instead, a goal defining 5–10% loss of their total weight is more realistic.
- *Assess possible barriers* to making lifestyle change and discuss solutions to overcome these barriers. Easy choices are realistic choices.

- *Define goals as precisely as possible*, for example, 'Walk 20 minutes a day' versus 'Take more physical exercise'.
- *Set up a timetable*, for example, 'Stop smoking on 1 January' versus 'Stop smoking when you feel you can'.
- When you wish to address more than one behavioural goal, design a *lifestyle modification plan* with concrete goals and a timetable for stepwise change.
- Include as many *practical elements* as possible and involve *peer support* (e.g. group meetings for physical exercise, heart sports groups, self-help groups).

Frequent monitoring and feedback

Numerous studies have shown that frequent monitoring and feedback are indispensable to lifestyle change interventions. The following behavioural techniques can be recommended:

- Self-monitoring of health behaviour
- Frequent feedback *by caregivers*.

Self-monitoring of behaviour, for example, use of a pedometer when attempting to increase physical activity levels allows an individual to monitor their progress daily and especially when combined with regular feedback from caregivers.

Feedback by caregivers should be provided regularly, for example, every 2 weeks in the first 3 months, with longer intervals thereafter. Keep in mind that changes in lifestyle can take up to 1 year to become stable, and that gradual change that is sustained is often more permanent than rapid change.

Specialist multidisciplinary prevention and rehabilitation programmes

Specialist programmes such as these are recommended for individuals at very high CVD risk or with clinically manifest CVD. They are also useful for patients whose barriers to lifestyle change are great because they are, for example, from a low socioeconomic status background, have little social support, and/or they have additional psychosocial risk factors (see also Chapter 17).

These interventions integrate the skills of *physicians, nurses, dieticians, experts in sports medicine*, and *psychologists*, and typically comprise the following elements:

- Education on healthy lifestyle and medical resources
- Supervised exercise programme
- Stress management training
- Counselling on other psychosocial risk factors than stress (e.g. depression and anxiety).

Their availability is dependent on the healthcare system in a country. There are many different service provision modalities and settings available. For example, in the United Kingdom, these programmes are ambulatory, whereas in other countries, such as Germany and Switzerland, programmes are more likely to be residential (see Chapters 20 and 21 where programme settings are discussed).

Effective interventions typically comprise 40–80 hours, divided over different time periods, ranging from daily interventions (4–5 hours) for 3–4 weeks, up to once or twice in a week (2–3 hours) for 1 year. There is evidence that more intense and longer interventions have better outcomes.

However, even after longer interventions, it is of major importance to ensure maintenance of behavioural change by regular monitoring and feedback.

More information on the specific content of these interventions is given in the 'Key reading'.

Reference

1. Perk J, De Backer G, Gohlke H, *et al*. European guidelines on cardiovascular disease prevention in clinical practice (version 2012). The Fifth Joint Task Force of the European Society of Cardiology and Other Societies on Cardiovascular Disease Prevention in Clinical Practice (constituted by representatives of nine societies and by invited experts). *Eur Heart J* 2012; 33:1635–701.

Key reading

Artinian NT, Fletcher GF, Mozaffarian D, *et al*. Interventions to promote physical activity and dietary lifestyle changes for cardiovascular risk reduction in adults. AHA scientific statement. *Circulation* 2010; 122:406–41.

General Medical Council. *Consent: Patients and Doctors Making Decisions Together*. London: GMC, 2008. http://www.gmc-uk.org/guidance/ethical_guidance/consent_guidance_index.asp

National Institute for Health and Clinical Excellence. *Behaviour Change: The Principles for Effective Interventions*. NICE Public Health Guidance 6. London: NICE, 2007. http://www.nice.org.uk/guidance/ph6

Rollnik S, Butler CC, Kinnersley P, *et al*. Motivational interviewing. *BMJ* 2010; 340:c1900.

Schwarzer R. Modelling health behaviour change: how to predict and modify the adoption and maintenance of health behaviours. *Appl Psychol Int Rev* 2008; 57:1–29.

Chapter 9

Engaging people in prevention initiatives

Key messages

- Understand that people rarely exist in isolation from a social network (such as their family).
- Use any opportunity to assess and advise on the risk status of family members of high-risk subjects.
- Remember that our role of health professionals and other caregivers is to help and not to impose.
- Recollect that social isolation can be a powerful risk factor and consider special efforts with such people.

Summary

- This chapter identifies social factors that influence lifestyle and cardiovascular risk. It considers benefits of involving families rather than individuals in isolation in preventive initiatives.

Considerations

- Partners (spouses) and first-degree relatives of patients with atherosclerotic disease are at higher risk of developing CVD than the general population.
- A family history of premature CVD may reflect a shared environment of risk factors, genetic influences, or both. The practical implications are the same—to try harder to help with risk factor management.
- Couples tend to share the same lifestyle and risk factors. Family aggregation of risk factors is partly determined by 'assortative mating'. In other words, individuals are more likely to select mates who have the same characteristics as themselves ('like marries like'). Following this selection, couples go on to share lifestyle habits over a prolonged period which may contribute to reinforcing the continuing presence of risk factors in both of them.
- People do not exist in isolation. They are part of a social network, which includes their close family, friends, and carers.

Table 9.1 Benefits of a family approach to CVD prevention and some cautions and considerations	
Benefits	Considerations
Positive social support from the family facilitates lifestyle changes, for example:

if the person in a household responsible for buying and cooking food is included in a preventive initiative, they will have a clear understanding of the principles of a cardioprotective diet

If family members are included in preventive initiatives, they will benefit and reduce their CVD risk

Families can discuss these initiatives together when they are at home and remind each other of their goals which may improve adherence with treatments and increase motivation

A truthful picture of lifestyle habits is more likely to emerge as a result of family members included in preventive initiatives

Lifestyle change is more likely to be sustained in the long term because of the continuing social support provided by the family members | Patients may not want their family members to be involved

People need their own space

Patients who live alone and cannot bring a family member with them may feel compromised |

- Family members living in the same household can support each other to make healthy lifestyle changes.
- The benefits and factors needing consideration in a family approach to prevention are summarized in Table 9.1.

Chapter 10

Treatment of tobacco dependence

Key messages

- Stimulating a quit attempt in patients who are smokers is an imperative. Always ask about smoking and offer support and follow-up
- Above all advise your patients that your job is to help them and not to judge them.
- Ambivalence about quitting is common in long-term dependent smokers—use motivational techniques to build self-efficacy.
- Always offer and encourage the use of pharmacotherapy to aid a quit attempt.

Summary

- This chapter covers practical strategies to motivate and support patients and families in becoming tobacco free. It includes information on how to use pharmacological products.

The challenge

Many of your patients with vascular disease or at high cardiovascular risk who smoke will have been smoking for years and have many attempts to stop behind them.
The challenge for you as a health professional is to stimulate a quit attempt:

- Smoking is a major cause of CVD which presents earlier in smokers compared to never smokers.
- Even very low tobacco consumption is harmful; there is no safe level.
- Smoking has a multiplicative interaction with other risk factors for CVD.
- The health benefits of quitting smoking are immediate.

Priorities in smoking cessation—the 'five A's'

- *Always* ask about smoking when you talk to your patients for the first time and validate their self-report with a biomarker (see Box 10.1).
- *Advise* those who are smoking to quit.
- *Assess* dependence on nicotine and motivation to quit in patients who are smokers.
- *Agree* on a strategy using counselling and pharmacology in those who are willing to quit.
- *Arrange* a programme of follow-up.

Use a breath carbon monoxide monitor to validate self-reported smoking status during a quit attempt:

- Accurate and reliable especially in heavy smokers
- Economical and non-invasive
- Gives an immediate result during a consultation
- Motivates recent quitters by demonstrating reduction in circulating carbon monoxide
- Picks up lapses early and so reduces likelihood of progression to full relapse.

A comprehensive assessment

Start off with a comprehensive assessment:

- *Smoking status*—always ask about smoking. Know who your smoking patients are!
- *Readiness to quit*—are they ready to quit now?
- *Motivation*—explore how ambivalent, how important, and how confident smokers feel about quitting. This may help to stimulate a new attempt to quit.
- *Dependence on nicotine*—how addicted is your patient to nicotine? This will help with tailoring the pharmacotherapy.
- *History of past quit attempts*—what has your patient tried in the past to quit? Do they associate it with success or failure?
- *Smoking in the family*—who else is smoking at home? What sort of social support can your patient expect? Will other family members try and quit too?
- *Psychological co-morbidities*—does your patient have a history of anxiety or depression? This may need close monitoring during a quit attempt because withdrawal from nicotine may precipitate depressive symptoms. However, in the long term, stopping smoking has been shown to improve mental health.

After many years of smoking and failed quit attempts, confidence to succeed in stopping may be low. Addiction creates ambivalence and an enormous barrier to making further stop smoking attempts.

Important imperatives in making success of a quit attempt:

- Offer support or refer to support
- Provide counselling—the higher the intensity, the higher the quit rate
- Provide effective pharmacotherapy—it increases success two- to threefold when combined with counselling.

Build self-efficacy:
- 'On a scale of 1–10, how important is it for you to quit?'
- 'Using the same scale, how confident are you that you can quit?'
- 'So why are you a … on the scale and not 10?'
- 'What would it take to move you from … to 10?'

Counselling

Assessing motivation to quit

- Most smokers want to stop but they rarely have plans to quit within the next 6 months.
- However, they may change their minds very quickly!
- An offer of support can stimulate a quit attempt.

Motivational interviewing techniques to explore and resolve ambivalence about quitting are shown in Boxes 10.2–10.5.

If a quit attempt is not possible …

Another option is to reduce smoking whilst using nicotine replacement therapy (NRT) (see Box 10.6). This strategy can lead to an eventual quit.

In smokers who are willing to reduce initially, and quit within 3 months, varenicline can increase successful quitting substantially. This can be achieved over a period of around 6 months (see Box 10.10).

See Chapter 8 for more information on how to use behavioural strategies to support lifestyle change.

Dependence

Tobacco dependence is often physical, mental, and social:
- Nicotine is as addictive as heroin or cocaine
- Smokers believe that cigarettes help them relax and relieves their stress

Express empathy:
- 'My job is to try to help you, not to yell at you.'
- 'I can understand that you have had difficulties in the past with tying to quit.'
- 'I can understand that you were difficult to get along with when you first stopped smoking, but this usually lasts for only 2 weeks or so. We could discuss what you can do to help during those 2 weeks, like taking medication that relieves these symptoms of withdrawal.'

Box 10.4 Motivational interviewing techniques: developing discrepancy

Discrepancy - explore the pros and cons of quitting
to the patient's core values and life goals

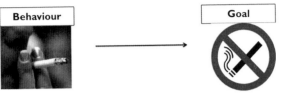

| Behaviour | | Goal |

'I think you know that smoking will help you to avoid
another heart attack or a new stent. What is stopping you
from quitting? What can you do to overcome the
difficulties?

- Stopping smoking can lead to perceptions of a loss of identity and exclusion from a social network
- Over the years, smoking becomes a real dependence that is difficult to kick.

Smokers may have feelings and beliefs that create barriers to quitting (see Fig. 10.1).

Measuring dependence on nicotine

Box 10.7 shows a simple tool for measuring dependence on nicotine. This simple test of nicotine dependency was developed from the Fagerstrom Test for Nicotine Dependence. A score of 4 or more indicates a high level of nicotine dependence, 2–3 = moderate dependence, and 0–1 points = light dependence.

Pharmacotherapy to support quit attempts

Therapies with the strongest evidence

- NRT
- Bupropion
- Varenicline.

All of these therapies reduce symptoms of withdrawal and craving which occur at the start of a quit smoking attempt. Boxes 10.8–10.10 include information on how to use these therapies effectively.

Box 10.5 Motivational interviewing techniques: avoiding argumentation

Avoid arguing with your patient:
- Help patients to find ways to succeed when they express reasons for not quitting.
- Keep the atmosphere relaxed.
- Offer help—not counterarguments.

Box 10.6 Using nicotine to assist reduction and a full quit attempt

Action on Smoking and Health (ASH) guidance—nicotine-assisted reduction to stop (licensing arrangements for NRT in the United Kingdom allow the use of this protocol):

- 0–6 weeks: cut down to 50% of initial consumption
- 6 weeks–9 months: continue to cut down and aim to stop completely by 6 months
- 6–9 months: stop smoking completely and continue to use NRT
- Within 12 months: stop using NRT by 12 months.

ASH recommendations:

- Prescriptions should be issued 2 weeks at a time.
- No repeat prescriptions should be issued during the cut-down period unless daily reduction is reported.
- Reduction should be validated with breath carbon monoxide readings.
- Once an individual decides to quit completely, calculate the NRT dose on the basis of initial tobacco consumption.

Duration of treatment—points to remember

- Prolonging the prescription of varenicline or NRT beyond the normal duration is acceptable.
- Do *not* worry about addiction to these therapies. It is ultimately preferable to a patient continuing or relapsing to smoking.
- Whichever product is in use, monitor tolerance and ensure the correct dose is taken. Do not be tempted to under-dose.

Other considerations

Harm reduction

- There may be some benefit in reducing harm by reducing exposure to tobacco in highly dependent smokers.
- Nicotine products that do not contain tobacco can be used to aid reduction in order to limit exposure to dangerous toxins contained in tobacco smoke.
- Trying to reduce smoking without treatment will lead to compensatory smoking (i.e. heavy drawing on each cigarette).
- Use of NRT for smoking reduction or temporary abstinence appears to be positively associated with subsequent attempts to quit smoking and abstinence among smokers in England.

Smokers may feel guilty and shameful about their smoking especially when they connect it with a cardiac event.	Self blame and a lack of success in quitting can lead to feelings of reduced confidence to quit.

Don't assume that your patient believes in the dangers of smoking. You may need to explore beliefs about smoking with your patients.

Figure 10.1 Feelings and beliefs about smoking.

Box 10.7 Heavy smoking index

How many cigarettes, on average, do you smoke per day?
- 1–10 (score 0)
- 11–20 (score 1)
- 21–30 (score 2)
- 31+ (score 3).

How soon after waking do you smoke your first cigarette?
- Within 5 minutes (score 3)
- 6–30 minutes (score 2)
- 31–60 minutes (score 1)
- 61+ minutes (score 0).

Box 10.8 Using nicotine replacement therapy

What is it?
- NRT contains small amounts of nicotine and is delivered via patches as a slow-release format, and via the oral, buccal, nasal, or sublingual mucosa more rapidly.

How does it work?
- NRT helps to relieve withdrawal symptoms by replacing nicotine.
- It comes in long- and short-acting forms, which makes it quite flexible.
- Using transdermal patches (long-acting) in conjunction with short-acting forms means that a quitter can have a background delivery of nicotine backed up by a short-acting delivery (e.g. from nasal spray, gum, or inhalator) when urges strike.

How is it used?
- Users can choose to use NRT either in one format or in combination formats.
- The most effective method is to use the long-acting format (transdermal patches) in combination with a short-acting format (e.g. gum, lozenges, or nasal or oral spray).
- Thus a background dose can be delivered over a 16-hour or 24-hour period backed up by quick bursts of nicotine delivered when a patient experiences urges to smoke (ad lib).
- NRT can be used to support smoking reduction where an abrupt attempt to quit is unrealistic (see Box 10.6).

Is it safe?
- NRT has been shown to be safe in patients with CVD.
- Whilst nicotine may have effects on the cardiovascular system, ultimately, NRT is safer than continuing to use tobacco.

Are there any side effects?
- Side effects from NRT are benign.
- They include skin irritation from the transdermal patch, which can be avoided by rotating the site of the patch, and oral and nasal irritation.

Box 10.9 Using bupropion

What is it?

- Bupropion is an antidepressant that has been found to be more effective than placebo for smoking cessation.
- Efficacy is not as impressive as varenicline or combination short- and long-acting NRT.

How does it work?

- Inhibits reuptake of dopamine, serotonin, and norepinephrine.
- Resulting increased bioavailability of these substances may help with relief from nicotine withdrawal.

How is it used?

- Start the treatment 1–2 weeks before the quit date.
- Increase the dose from 150 mg every morning for 6 days to 150 mg twice daily.
- Continue the treatment for between 7 and 9 weeks.

Is it safe?

- Safe for use in patients with vascular disease and in those who are at high cardiovascular risk.
- Associated with an increased risk of seizure.
- Contraindications including epilepsy, anorexia, bulimia, bipolar disease, and severe liver cirrhosis.

Are there any side effects?

- Dry mouth
- Insomnia
- Tremor
- Taste or visual disturbance.

- Evidence for e-cigarettes for smoking reduction and cessation is increasing. Some evidence indicates that e-cigarettes may be as effective as NRT but more data are needed.

Weight gain

- Weight gain is common after stopping smoking. People gain an average of 4–5 kg over a year.
- A minority gain a lot more (up to 12 kg) and a few gain no weight at all.
- Weight gain can have an adverse effect on the cardiovascular risk profile.
- Quitting smoking has immediate benefits to health and so should be prioritized above weight control.
- A tailored programme of individualized dietary and physical activity support during smoking cessation may minimize weight gain.

| Box 10.10 Using varenicline |

What is it?
- Nicotinic partial receptor agonist specially developed to help smoking cessation.

How does it work?
- Provides relief from withdrawal and reduces reward from smoking by binding to and partially stimulating the $\alpha 4\beta 2$ nicotinic receptor in the brain.

How is it used?
- It is usual to set a quit date 8 days ahead; however, some smokers need longer. In quitters allowed up to 5 weeks to set a date, the median date set was around 2 weeks.
- Start 0.5 mg dose once daily. Continue at this dose for the first 3 days.
- On day 4, up-titrate to 0.5 mg twice daily for 4 days.
- From day 8, up-titrate to 1 mg twice daily for 12 weeks.
- If more than several weeks pass before the patient quits, consider a second 12-week course, which has been shown to improve quit rates in smokers who quit late into their first course.
- Varenicline has also been shown to be helpful for retreatment in people who used it previously.

Is it safe?
- Shown to be safe for patients with stable CVD.
- Does not appear to be associated with neuropsychiatric harm in comparison with placebo.
- Shown to be effective and safe in smokers who are under effective treatment for depression or who have suffered in the past with major depression.
- Some monitoring is still recommended regarding psychological state of smokers taking varenicline.

Are there any side effects?
- 30% experience nausea which is helped by taking varenicline straight after eating food or drinking 1–2 glasses of water. Antiemetics may be prescribed if required.
- Vivid dreams: usually wears off after 2–3 weeks.
- Some may experience difficulty falling asleep and/or waking early but this usually subsides after 2–3 weeks.

Smoking cessation in hospitalized patients with ACS

Varenicline was recently shown to be effective for cessation in smokers hospitalized with ACS. There was no increase in adverse or major cardiovascular events within 30 days of discontinuation of the drug.

Bupropion has not demonstrated efficacy in this group of high risk patients, and evidence for NRT in this area is very limited.

Key reading

Aubin HJ, Farley A, Lycett, D, et al. Weight gain in smokers after quitting cigarettes: meta-analysis. *BMJ* 2012; 345:e4439.

Cahill K, Stevens S, Perera R, et al. Pharmacological interventions for smoking cessation: an overview and network meta-analysis. *Cochrane Database Syst Rev* 2013; 5:CD009329.

Ebbert JO et al. Effect of varenicline on smoking reduction: a randomised clinical trial. *JAMA* 2015; 313:687–94.

Eisenberg MJ et al. Varenicline for smoking cessation in hospitalised patients with acute coronary syndrome. *Circulation* 2015. E pub ahead of print.

Heatherton TF, Kozlowski LT, Frecker RC et al. The Fagerstrom Test for Nicotine Dependence: a revision of the Fagerstrom Tolerance Questionnaire. *Br J Addict* 1991; 86:1119–27.

Jennings C, Kotseva K, De Bacquer D, et al. Effectiveness of a preventive cardiology programme for high CVD risk persistent smokers: the EUROACTION PLUS varenicline trial. *Eur Heart J* 2014; 35:1411–20.

National Institute for Health and Care Excellence. Tobacco: harm-reduction approaches to smoking. NICE Public Health Guidance 45. London: NICE, 2013. http://www.nice.org.uk/guidance/ph45

Chapter 11

Diet and weight: major lifestyle challenges

Key messages

- A detailed dietary assessment is essential to tailoring of dietary advice.
- Focus on fresh, unprocessed food as far as possible.
- Understanding dietary patterns rather than single nutrient intake is important.
- Changing from unhealthy eating patterns to a cardioprotective diet can make an important contribution to managing biomedical risk factors and reducing cardiovascular risk.
- Obesity is a global epidemic with central obesity being a major driver of metabolic abnormalities associated with cardiovascular risk.
- Obesity occurs when energy intake exceeds energy expenditure in everyday eating habits.
- Obesity occurs as a result of a complex interplay of behavioural and societal factors.
- Anthropometric measurements form an important part of a comprehensive cardiovascular assessment.
- Obese people can benefit significantly from losing as little as 10% of their body weight.
- Reducing calorie intake can be achieved not only by reducing food intake but also by altering the balance of food groups in the diet and swapping unhealthy for healthier options.

Summary

- This chapter covers practical methodologies for assessing dietary habits in individuals and advising on and facilitating healthy dietary changes.
- It also describes practical methodologies for taking anthropometric measurements and managing weight in individuals and families.

Diet

Assessment of dietary habits

Dietary intake has many different influences. These influences will vary between individuals. Developing an understanding of these influences is essential to complete a detailed and accurate assessment.

Therefore, the following factors should be addressed and taken into consideration.

Identification of assessment purpose

- Assess overall dietary balance and pattern
- Identify level of consumption of specific or groups of foods
- Obtain a quantitative estimate of energy and/or nutrient intake
- Identify nutritional deficiencies or surpluses
- Identify food-related symptoms
- Assess risk of malnutrition or overeating/overdrinking
- Monitor adherence to dietary advice.

When trying to establish a typical dietary intake of a person/family, it is essential to consider possible influences that may affect food choice. This will enable the health professional to establish daily variation in terms of both frequency and quantity.

Factors affecting food choices

- Cultural, religious, or ethical beliefs
- Psychological (rewarding, punishing, or comfort eating)
- Appetite level, taste preferences
- Financial issues/facilities available
- Lifestyle/work hours and commitments (e.g. shift work, business travel/entertaining, and type of work hence availability of access to food/beverages)
- Difference between weekdays and weekends
- Social conventions/how food is eaten (e.g. in front of TV, sat as a family at a table, and 'on the move')
- Meals taken outside of the home
- Family/peer group pressures
- Advertising
- Knowledge/beliefs about food and diet
- Previous advice or previous diet attempts including weight history.

Readiness to change

Changing dietary habits of a lifetime can be very difficult. All subjects should be assessed for their readiness and motivation to change. To be beneficial, dietary changes need to be long term. Therefore all suggested changes should be realistic and achievable. For more information on assessing motivation and readiness to change, see Chapter 8.

Household influences

The dynamics of any household has a strong influence on the dietary habits of the people living within that house. Identification and collaboration with the person who is in charge of the food purchasing and food preparation is essential to improve outcome and long-term dietary change.

Dietary assessment methods

Dietary habits are complex and very variable, leading to challenges in their measurement. Therefore the tools used need to be selected carefully. Not only is it essential to establish what is consumed, it is also important to gain an insight into the processes and feelings the family go through for food and drink selection, preparation, and consumption.

People are often sensitive about what they eat and drink. This can lead to reluctance and underestimation of what they perceive as 'bad' foods and overestimation of 'good' foods. To reduce this possible error it is important to ask open, indirect, and non-leading questions:

Closed question: Do you have milk in coffee?

Open question: How do you have your coffee?

Direct question: How much butter do you use?

Indirect question: How long does a pack of butter last you?

Leading question: What do you have for breakfast?

Non-leading: What would be the first thing you would eat or drink in the morning?

Obtaining dietary information with these methods of questioning in mind is essential. The quality of dietary modification advice relies completely on the quality and accuracy of the data collected in the assessment.

Recall methods

Food frequency questionnaire Collection of data on the frequency a food or drink item is consumed and the amount eaten on each sitting. This is either interview led or completed by the participant.

24-hour recall Interview-led recall collects information about the previous day's intake. Foods and drinks are described and portions estimated. Multiple days improve precision.

Diet history Interview-led, obtaining detailed information about usual foods and drinks consumed. Portion sizes, food preparation methods, and food frequency information are also collected.

Mediterranean diet score This is a 9- or 14-point score.[1] All elements of the Mediterranean diet are included and a point is scored for adherence to each element. An increase of 2 points in this score is associated with a 9% reduction in cardiovascular risk (Table 11.1).

Table 11.1 Mediterranean dietary score tool	
Question	Yes/No
Is olive oil the main culinary fat used?	
Are ≥4 tablespoons of olive oil used each day?	
Are ≥2 servings (of 200 g each) of vegetables eaten each day?	
Are ≥3 servings (of 80 g each) of fruit eaten each day?	
Is <1 serving (100–150 g) of red meat/hamburgers/other meat products eaten each day?	
Is <1 serving (12 g) of butter, margarine, or cream eaten each day?	
Is <1 serving (330 mL) of sweet or sugar-sweetened carbonated beverages consumed each day?	
Are ≥3 glasses (of 125 mL) of wine consumed each week?	
Are ≥3 servings (of 150 g) of legumes eaten each week?	
Are ≥3 servings (of 100–150 g) of fish or (200 g) seafood eaten each week?	
Are <3 servings of commercial sweets/pastries eaten each week?	
Is ≥1 serving (50 g) of nuts consumed each week?	
Is chicken, turkey, or rabbit routinely eaten instead of veal, pork, hamburger, or sausages?	
Are pasta, vegetable, or rice dishes flavoured with garlic, tomato, leek, or onion eaten ≥2 times a week?	
TOTAL SCORE (total number of 'yes' answers)	

Record methods

- *Diet records/diaries*: the participant records all that is eaten and drunk during a given period, most commonly 3 or 7 days. The portions are described either in household measures, weighed, in average portions, from photographs, or in pack sizes.
- *Checklist record*: this is a list of food. Each time a participant eats a food he or she ticks it off the list and records the portion size consumed.

Portion size estimation

- It is essential to quantify the amount of food eaten but this is often difficult to quantify.
- Weighing each food item is the most accurate way although it is very labour intensive.
- Participant perception of what equals an average portion may vary.
- Underestimation of portion size is common, especially of those foods that are perceived to be bad.
- The use of photographs showing a variety of portions sizes can improve estimation.

24-hour recall methodology

In clinical practice, 24-hour recall and diet histories are the most frequently used methods. A standardized method of completing a 24-hour recall in shown in the following sections; a similar method can be applied to a diet history methodology.

Triple-pass method

Aim: to provide a complete record of all food and drink on the previous day between midnight and midnight.

The 24-hour recall is collected in three phases (triple-pass):[2]

1. A quick list of foods eaten or drunk

- Ask subjects to report everything that they had to eat or drink on the previous day between midnight and midnight.
- Do not interrupt.
- At the end of the recall, invite subjects to add any additional items not initially recalled.

2. Collection of detailed information of the items in the quick list

- For each item of food, ask the subjects to provide additional detail.
- Use open questioning.

- Ask subjects to describe and quantify food in a consistent way:
  - Type (salmon, lamb, cabbage, rice, potatoes)
  - State of food (canned, frozen, fresh)
  - Cut of food (fillet, whole, slice, small pieces)
  - Cooking method (fried, roasted, boiled, steamed)
  - Amount eaten.
- Foods likely to be eaten in combination with other items should be prompted for:
  - For example, milk in coffee
  - Sandwiches (fillings and bread)
  - Pasta and salad.
- The quantity consumed should be based on household measures, food photographs, or named products.
  - For example, amount eaten =1 apple, 2 slices of meat, 2 tablespoons, 1 cup.

3. A recall review

- Review all the food eaten and drunk.
- Prompt for any additional eating occasions or foods possibly consumed and clarify any ambiguities (portion sizes, food eaten).

- *Forgotten foods*—ask specific questions on the following:
  - Soft drinks
  - Alcoholic drinks
  - Sweets/chocolate/confectionery
  - Crisps/nuts/other snacks
  - Dressings/sauces
  - Salt/pepper
  - Dietary supplements.

Validation of assessment methods

All types of dietary assessments on free-living subjects rely to varying extents on the ability of the subject to record or recall their intake. This provides a source of error, either through under- or over-reporting or falsifications. Research has shown, for example, that those who are obese, female, or trying to lose weight will under-report their intake.

The best way to validate intake is by using biomarkers. Table 11.2 shows possible different biomarkers for different nutrients. These are often expensive, invasive, time-consuming, and depend on the precision of the assays, so are rarely completed in clinical practice.

Cardioprotective dietary patterns

Research into dietary habits now focuses on whole dietary patterns rather than individual nutrients, which are rarely consumed in isolation.

A large variation in dietary patterns exists across Europe. This variation has been associated with differences in cardiovascular mortality rates between northern and southern Europe.[3] It is likely that that the 'Mediterranean diet' consumed in the southern parts of Europe largely explains this difference.

Mediterranean diet

Adherence to a Mediterranean diet, assessed using the Mediterranean diet score (see Table 11.1), is associated with reduced risk. A change of 2 in the score has been shown to reduce cardiovascular incidence and mortality by 9%. This has recently been supported by a RCT (PREDIMED) which showed a reduction in CVD events in high-risk patients when following a Mediterranean diet.[4]

Table 11.2 Examples of biomarkers for reported nutrient validation

Nutrient	Possible biomarker
Energy intake	Doubly labelled water
Protein	24-hour nitrogen excretion in urine
Omega-3 fatty acids	Levels in adipose tissue or blood
Sodium and potassium	24-hour sodium and potassium excretion in urine
Antioxidants	Levels in plasma

DASH diet

The DASH diet, based on the research studies 'Dietary Approaches to stop Hypertension', is rich in fruit and vegetables and low in fat and non-fat dairy. It places great emphasis on wholegrains and has less refined grains than the typical Western diet. It is rich in potassium, calcium, magnesium, and fibre but low in sodium. RCTs have shown the beneficial effect the diet has on cardiovascular risk factors.

Portfolio diet

The portfolio diet combines the dietary advice that are common to the major randomized control trials. The combined effect showed a 30% reduction in LDL-C under controlled conditions (equivalent to lovastatin).[5] Longer-term effects over 1 year in free-living, compliant, and motivated subjects showed a 20% reduction in LDL.[6] There were no data for CVD events or mortality.

Table 11.3 shows a comparison of three different cardioprotective dietary patterns.

European dietary recommendations

The European recommendations are in-line with a Mediterranean dietary pattern (see Box 11.1).

Table 11.3 Comparison of three different cardioprotective dietary patterns

	Mediterranean diet	DASH diet	Portfolio diet
8–10 portions of fruit and vegetables	✓	✓	✓
>3 portions of wholegrains per day (20 g/day)	✓	✓	✓
Low saturated fat	✓	✓	✓
High unsaturated fat	✓	✓	✓
Fish >2/week	✓	✓	
Oily fish >1/week	✓	✓	
Fresh rather than processed foods	✓	✓	✓
Moderate alcohol intake	✓		
Nuts/seeds legumes (30 g/day)	✓	✓	✓
Stanol/sterol esters (2 g/day)			✓
Soya products (50 g/day)			✓
Low-fat dairy options <2 per day	✓	✓	✓
Reduced salt intake	✓	✓	✓

Box 11.1 European dietary recommendations

- Saturated fatty acids to account for less than 10% of total energy intake, through replacement by polyunsaturated fatty acids
- Trans-unsaturated fatty acids: as little as possible, preferably no intake from processed food, and 1% of total energy intake from natural origin.
- Less than 5 g of salt per day
- 30–45 g of fibre per day, from wholegrain products, fruits, and vegetables
- 200 g of fruit per day (2–3 servings)
- 200 g of vegetables per day (2–3 servings)
- Fish at least twice a week, one of which to be oily fish
- Consumption of alcoholic beverages should be limited to two glasses per day (20 g/day of alcohol) for men and one glass per day (10 g/day of alcohol) for women
- Energy intake should be limited to the amount of energy needed to maintain (or obtain) a healthy weight (i.e. a BMI <25 kg/m^2)
- In general when following the rules for a healthy diet, no dietary supplements are needed.

Fats

A cardioprotective diet is quite high in fat but the ratio of saturated to unsaturated is what appears to help prevent CVD. It is often misconceived that a cardioprotective diet is low in fat. Fat is an essential part of the diet, required for:

- providing essential fatty acids
- acting as a carrier for fat-soluble vitamins (A, D, E, and K) and antioxidants
- acting as a protective layer around organs
- essential structural, storage, and metabolic functions
- improving food flavour and palatability
- growth and development
- energy for cells through oxidation.

Fat is usually grouped into four main types depending on its structure:

- Saturated fatty acid (SFA)
- Monounsaturated fatty acid (MUFA)
- Polyunsaturated fatty acid (PUFA):
  - Omega-3 PUFA
  - Omega-6 PUFA
- Trans fatty acid (TFA).

Their sources and effects on CVD risk factors are listed in Table 11.4.

Practical tips to improve fat intake

- Avoid obvious high sources of SFA and TFA (visible fat, creamy/cheese sauces, pastry, cakes, and biscuits).
- Increase the use of unsaturated fats and use nuts and seeds as a healthy snack.

Table 11.4 Sources of fatty acids and their effects on CVD risk

Type of fat (fatty acid)	Where it is found	Effect on CVD risk factors
SFA (palmitic acid, stearic acid)	Animal products: meat fat, cheese, cream, butter, dripping, pastry, ghee. Plant products: coconut, palm oil	Increases LDL. Increases HDL. Enhances atherosclerosis development
MUFA Omega-9 (oleic acid)	Olive oil. Rapeseed oil. Ground nut (peanut) oil. Nuts and seeds (almonds, hazelnuts, pecan, macadamia). Avocado	Reduces TC and LDL-C cholesterol when substituting saturated fat. Small increase in HDL. Less risk of lipid peroxidation than polyunsaturated fat
PUFA Omega 3 (alpha-linolenic acid, eicosapentaenoic acid (EPA), docosahexaenoic acid (DHA))	Oils: canola/rapeseed, flaxseed. Oily fish: mackerel, salmon, sardines, trout, pilchards, herrings. Enriched products: eggs, milk, yogurt	Minimal effect on blood cholesterol. Very high doses reduces TGs. Antithrombotic, antiarrhythmic, and anti-inflammatory effect
PUFA Omega-6 (linoleic acid, arachidonic acid)	Oils: sunflower, safflower, corn, walnut, and soybean	Reduces LDL and TC. Increases HDL slightly. Enhances lipid peroxidation and free radical production
TFA (partially hydrogenated fatty acids)	Dairy products, cakes, biscuits, processed foods, deep-fried fast foods	Increases LDL. Increases TC. Decreases HDL. Enhances atherosclerosis development

- Be vigilant about removing fat in the cooking process.
- Reduced the amount of fat added to cooking by measuring it out.
- Try not to fry—steam, boil, microwave, or bake instead.
- Choose leaner meats and leaner cuts of meat.
- Choose lower-fat options.
- Change the proportions on your plate so you have more vegetables than protein or carbohydrate.

Fish oils

Previously, epidemiological and clinical evidence suggested that increased intake of omega-3 fatty acids, particularly EPA and DHA, protected against mortality from CAD.[7,8] These fatty acids are naturally found in high quantities in oily fish. Although earlier trials (DART trial and GISSI-P trial)[9,10] have shown a protective effect of omega-3 fatty acids in MI patients, in these studies they were not optimally medically treated like they are now. More recent studies have thus not been able to replicate the large protective effect previously seen (GISSI-HF).[11] In this study, the PUFA supplements only provided a small additional benefit on top of standard optimal treatment.

As there is no evidence of harm, oily fish should still be included in a cardioprotective diet but the higher intake emphasized in previous guidelines has now changed.

Fruit and vegetables

A variety of fruit and vegetables are an essential part of the cardioprotective diet.

They are beneficial for the prevention of many chronic diseases including heart disease as they are:

- high in soluble fibre and therefore have a low glycaemic index
- high in antioxidants, folic acid, and potassium
- low in fat and calories.

How does this reduce risk?

- Reduces cholesterol levels by reducing fat absorption
- Protects against formation of oxidized LDL
- Protects against free radicals
- Reduces homocysteine levels
- Reduces BP
- Helps with weight management
- Improves gut transit time
- Improves glycaemic control especially in diabetics.

Recommended intake

- Minimum of 5 portions each day but aim for 8–10 portions (see Box 11.2)
- This can be a combination of fruit and vegetable but tipping the balance in favour of vegetables is better
- Try to have a variety of colours to get different vitamins and minerals
- Fresh, frozen, or tinned in natural juices is ok
- Fruit juice/smoothies only count as 1 portion
- Potatoes do not count.

Are there any fruits and vegetables that should be avoided?

The only one to avoid is grapefruit/grapefruit juice when certain statins have been prescribed—check the medication information leaflet.

Vitamin supplements

An adequate vitamin and mineral intake is ensured in the presence of varied and balanced nutrition. High doses of supplements have been associated with harmful effects.

Carbohydrate, wholegrains, and fibre

Carbohydrates

Carbohydrates provide a major source of energy and are derived from plant foods. They are often divided into two groups although this divide is not clear-cut:

- Digestible carbohydrate (associated with a postprandial rise in blood glucose) is broken down to produce glucose, which is essential for brain and body tissue function.

Box 11.2 Portion sizes of fruit and vegetables

Diet

Fruit

- Apricot, dried: 3 whole
- Apricot, fresh: 3 apricots
- Banana, fresh: 1 medium banana
- Blueberries: 2 handfuls (4 heaped tablespoons)
- Clementines: 2 clementines
- Fruit juice: 1 × 150 mL glass
- Fruit salad, canned: 3 heaped tablespoons
- Fruit smoothie: 1 × 150 mL glass
- Grapes: 1 handful
- Mango: 5 × 5 cm slices
- Melon: 1 slice (5 cm slice)
- Mixed fruit, dried: 1 heaped tablespoon
- Nectarine/peach: 1 nectarine
- Orange: 1 orange
- Pear, canned: 2 halves or 7 slices
- Pineapple, canned: 2 rings or 12 chunks
- Plum: 2 medium plums
- Prune, canned: 6 prunes
- Strawberry, fresh: 7 strawberries
- Sultanas: 1 heaped tablespoon.

Vegetables

- Asparagus, fresh: 5 spears
- Aubergine: 1/3 aubergine
- Beans, broad/butter/kidney cooked: 3 heaped tablespoons
- Beansprouts, fresh: 2 handfuls
- Beetroot, bottled: 3 'baby' whole or 7 slices
- Broccoli: 2 spears
- Brussel sprouts: 8 Brussel sprouts
- Carrots, fresh/canned slices: 3 heaped tablespoons
- Cauliflower: 8 florets
- Celery: 3 sticks
- Leeks: 1 leek (white portion only)
- Lentils: 3 tablespoons
- Lettuce (mixed leaves): 1 cereal bowl
- Mixed vegetables, frozen: 3 tablespoons
- Onion, fresh: 1 medium onion

- Parsnips: 1 large parsnip
- Peas, canned/fresh/frozen: 3 heaped tablespoons
- Spinach, cooked: 2 heaped tablespoons
- Spring greens, cooked: 4 heaped tablespoons
- Tomato, fresh: 1 medium, 7 cherry.

- Non-digestible carbohydrates (not associated with a postprandial rise in blood glucose) are important to gastrointestinal function. It is thought that these may be absorbed in the colon following fermentation.

Glycaemic index

The glycaemic index (GI) describes the effect that different carbohydrates have on glucose levels. Low GI carbohydrates produce only small fluctuations in our blood glucose and insulin levels. This is important for long-term health and reducing the risk of heart disease and diabetes (see Table 11.5).

The GI of a food will also vary depending on how it is cooked, processed, and prepared (ingredients), and its ripeness. It is also rare for foods to be eaten in isolation, therefore it is important to think of the glycaemic load—this is the effect on postprandial glucose that the whole meal will have, rather than the individual foods, for example, combining a high-GI food with a low-GI food will lead to a medium-GI load (e.g. jacket potato and baked beans).

Table 11.5 Glycaemic index of different food groups			
Food	Low GI	Medium GI	High GI
Rice	Basmati	Brown/white	
Bread	Wholegrain, granary	Pitta, muffin, croissant	Baguette, bagel, wholemeal
Cereals	Oat based (e.g. porridge, muesli), bran rich	Cereal bars	Wheat or maize based (e.g. cornflakes, Weetabix®)
Potatoes	New potatoes in their skins	Boiled old potatoes, chips	Mashed, instant, jacket potatoes
Fruit	Most fruits	Dried fruit, banana, pineapple	Fruit juice, watermelon, lychees
Vegetables	All green and salad vegetables, carrots, yam	Sweet potato, sweetcorn, beetroot	Pumpkin, parsnips
Dairy foods	Plain yoghurt, milk		Flavoured yoghurt
Sugar	Fructose	Sucrose, honey	Glucose, Lucozade®

Benefits of a low GI diet
- Weight management—reduces hunger and keeps you feeling fuller for longer
- Increases insulin sensitivity
- Improves diabetes control
- Reduces the risk of heart disease
- Improves lipid profiles
- Helps manage the symptoms of polycystic ovary syndrome.

Wholegrains

- Wholegrain refers to the unrefined, intact grain containing the bran, germ, and endosperm. Wholegrains include whole oats.
- Meta-analysis evidence from 11 prospective cohort studies has shown a 19% reduction in the risk of developing CHD is associated with greater wholegrain consumption.[12]
- At least three servings a day of wholegrain to replace refined grain varieties of food is typically recommended.

Dietary fibre

- There is an inverse relationship between fibre intake and CVD risk. A 7 g increase in fibre intake is related to a 7% reduction in cardiovascular risk. Vegetable fibre appears to be more beneficial than fibre from fruit or cereal sources.[13]
- Soluble fibre helps to improve lipid profiles by reducing LDL-C.
- Ideal intake is 25–30 g of total dietary fibre, which includes 7–13 g of soluble fibre (fibre from oat bran, beta-glucan, and psyllium).
- Confounding factors—most people who have a high-fibre diet also have a healthier lifestyle (e.g. low saturated fat intake, more exercise, and being non-smokers), and consequently lower BMI, BP, and TG levels.

Ways to increase fibre intake
- Choose wholegrain products
- Use wholemeal flour or use half white, half brown
- Eat the skins on fruit and vegetables
- Add fruit, nuts, and seeds to cereals and salads
- Do not mash or blend fruit and vegetables.
See Table 11.6.

Sugars and sweeteners

Sugar

- Sugar has very little nutritional value.
- Globally, sugar intake has increased from:
  - changes in processed food formulation to reduce fat and to ensure the product remains palatable
  - increased intake of sugar-sweetened beverages (SSBs).

Table 11.6 Types of fibre, their role in prevention, and their sources		
Type	Role	Sources
Soluble fibre	Reduces postprandial lipid and glucose absorption	Pulses, beans, oats, fruit, and vegetables
Insoluble fibre	Increases stool weight and transit time	Bran, potato skins, seeds, wholemeal products, and nuts
Resistant starch	Fermentation produces short-chain fatty acids	Modified starch, potato, green banana, rice, and bread
Prebiotics, fructo-oligosaccharides, and fructans	Equilibrates gut flora Laxation Fermentation produces short-chain fatty acids	Functional foods—added to products Leeks, bananas, and onions
Indigestible animal products	Cholesterol lowering	Seafood shells
Phytates	Reduces absorption of calcium, zinc, and iron. Also thought to protect against cancer due to the effect of reduced absorption of iron to reduce cell growth	Legumes, grains, and soybeans

This increased intake of SSBs tracks the rising rates of obesity, this may be due to the limited effect SSBs have on satiety.

Cohort studies suggest an independent association of SSBs with CVD. A 35% higher risk of developing CHD in women has been associated with drinking two SSBs a day compared with one a month.[14] A 20% higher relative risk of CHD in men has been associated with daily consumption compared with never consuming them.[15]

Sweeteners

Artificial sweeteners have no nutritional value and are sweeter than sugar. They may be useful in diabetic and overweight patients.

There are four main types commonly used in food products and drinks:

- Aspartame (Nutraswee™)
- Saccharin
- Acesulfame potassium (acesulfame K)
- Cyclamates.

These are available in tablet, liquid, and sprinkle form for use at home. Sorbitol and xylitol are alcohol sweeteners and contain calories. In large amounts they can cause osmotic diarrhoea and are not routinely recommended.

Nuts

- Nuts are high in protein, unsaturated fats, and fibre.
- Cohort studies show a 30% reduction in developing CHD.[12]
- Meta-analysis of 25 RCTs found a daily 67 g serving of nuts, significantly reduced TC, LDL-C, and TC:HDL ratio. TG levels were also reduced.

- The effects of nut consumption were dose related.
- Different types of nuts had similar effects on blood lipid levels. Although the greatest benefit is in those with a high LDL-C and low BMI.[16]
- Nuts are high in calories, however the evidence does not suggest increases in body weight. This is thought mainly to be due to dietary compensation.[17]
- Caution should be taken in those with a less competent appetite regulation or on a calorie controlled diet.
- A 60 g serving of mixed nuts contains ~400 kcal.
- Daily consumption can be recommended and can include a variety of nuts (e.g. almonds, walnuts, hazelnuts, pecans, pistachios, macadamias, and peanuts).
- Nuts should be unsalted and not covered in honey or other flavourings.

Protein

Proteins are comprised of amino acids. They are the building blocks of the body to manage metabolism and organ function. There are three types of amino acids:

- Essential—not synthesized by the body so must be present in the diet
- Non-essential—readily synthesized by the body.
- Conditionally essential—can be synthesized but may be needed from the diet under certain circumstances.

Protein requirements

- Healthy adult: 0.75–0.83 g protein/kg ideal body weight/day.
- The average intake in the United Kingdom is usually well above this level.
- During pregnancy or lactation, requirements increase.

Protein sources

Protein is obtained from both animal (meat, fish, poultry, and eggs) and plant (pulses, legumes, soya, nuts, and beans) sources.

Most people in the United Kingdom and Europe get the majority of their protein from animal sources. These sources are often associated with excessive saturated fat and therefore can be detrimental to prevention of CVD.

Ways to reduce saturated fat from protein sources

- Remove all visible fat prior to cooking (including chicken skin)
- Choose lean cuts of meat
- Choose low-fat dairy options
- Try not to fry—poach, grill, or bake instead.

Soy protein

Including soy protein in the diet may beneficial for reducing CVD risk.
Possible benefits of replacing lean meat with soy protein:

- Decreases TC, LDL, and TGs without altering HDL
- May be protective against LDL oxidation susceptibility.

Observations from the Anderson trial[18] suggest that the daily consumption of 31–47 g of soy protein can significantly decrease serum cholesterol and LDL-C (ingestion of 25 or 50 g of soy protein/day was estimated to decrease serum cholesterol concentration by 0.23 mmol/L and 0.45 mmol/L respectively). An intake of more than 30 g of soy protein/day can be achieved by consuming 2–3 servings of soy products daily:

- 226 g soy milk ≡ 4–10 g protein
- 113 g tofu ≡ 8–13 g protein
- 28 g soy flour ≡ 10–13 g protein
- 113 g textured protein ≡ 11 g protein
- 90 g meat analogue ≡ 18 g protein.

Alcohol

Alcohol is not an essential nutrient. The relationship between alcohol and total mortality has a U or J shape. Non-drinkers have a slightly higher risk than moderate drinkers. This does not mean that non-drinkers should be encouraged to start drinking. Recommended safe intakes are shown in Box 11.3.

Possible benefits of alcohol

- Increases HDL
- Inhibition of platelet aggregation.

Observational studies suggest that wine does not appear to be any more beneficial than any other type of alcohol.[19]

Possible problems with high alcohol intake (>3 units/day for women; >4 units/day for men)

- Can be addictive
- High in calories (7 kcal/g)
- Detrimental to the liver
- Raises BP
- Raises TGs
- Induces poor blood sugar control in diabetics
- Binge drinking can adversely affect cardiac muscle.

Optimum consumption is lower for women than for men because of enzymatic differences in alcohol metabolism between women and men.

Mixer drinks should be sugar free. Consumption of low-carbohydrate beers and 'low-alcohol' drinks are not preferential because of their higher alcohol and energy content.

Box 11.3 Recommended safe intake of alcohol for people at risk of CVD

- Men: maximum 10–30 g ethanol/day (1–3 units/day)
- Women: maximum 10–20 g ethanol/day (1–2 units/day).

NB Most people underestimate their alcohol intake. It has also been observed that those who drink more often have a higher intake of salt, which in turn could affect their BP. Therefore, each case should be considered individually.

Ways to reduce alcohol intake

- Drink half pints rather than pints.
- Put your drink down in between sips and move to your non-hand drinking side.
- Be aware of alcohol content in drinks (see Table 11.7).
- Measure drinks out at home and use smaller glasses.
- Have soft drinks on the table.

Salt

Sodium is an essential nutrient. Its balance in the body is maintained by effective homeostatic mechanisms. It is essential for regulation of fluid balance, BP, and transmembrane gradients. Chloride is also important for fluid balance, and gastric and intestinal secretions. Most intake is from common salt and is eaten in excess of requirements.

- Recommended intake is less than 5 g/day.
- In the United Kingdom and Europe, the average intake is ~9 g/day; 75% of this is estimated to come from processed foods.
- Effect of a high salt intake: increases BP and consequently CVD risk.

Table 11.7 Alcohol content in different drinks			
Drink	Alcohol by volume	Measure	Number of units (grams)
Beers, lagers, and cider	3–5%	250 mL (1/2 pint)	0.75–1.25 (7.5–12.5)
		500 mL (1 pint)	1.5–2.5 (15–25)
	6–8%	250 mL (1/2 pint)	1.5–2.0 (15–20)
		500 mL (1 pint)	3.0–4.0 (30–40)
Wine	9–11%	Small glass (125 mL)	1.0–1.4 (10–14)
		Medium glass (175 mL)	1.6–2.0 (16–20)
		Large glass (250 mL)	2.25–2.75 (22.5–27.5)
		1 bottle	6.75–8.25 (67.5–82.5)
	12–14%	Small glass (125 mL)	1.5–1.75 (15–17.5)
		Medium glass (175 mL)	2.1–2.45 (21–24.5)
		Large glass (250 mL)	3.0–3.5 (30–35)
		1 bottle	9.0–10.5 (90–105)
Fortified wine, e.g. sherry/port	16%	50 mL glass	0.8 (8.0)
Spirits, e.g. vodka/gin	40%	25 mL	1.0 (10)

Box 11.4 Food sources high in salt

- Ready-made meals
- Bread and cereals
- Cheese
- Tinned or packet soups and sauces
- Salted snacks—crisps, nuts
- Sausages, pies, and pâté
- Smoked meat with added salt
- Stock cubes, meat and vegetable extracts, soya sauce, and marmite.

- Benefits of lowering salt intake: reduces BP and CVD risk (salt reduction of 3 g/day could lead to a 3.5 mmHg reduction in SBP).

Practical advice to lower salt intake

- Discourage use of salt at the table or in cooking.
- Discourage consumption of foods with a high salt content (see Box 11.4).
- Encourage use of alternative ingredients to flavour foods (see Box 11.5).
- Do not recommend salt substitutes.

Functional foods

Definition

'Functional foods' are foods or dietary components that may provide a health benefit beyond basic nutrition. Examples can include fruits and vegetables, wholegrains, fortified or enhanced foods and beverages, and some dietary supplements. Biologically active components in functional foods may impart health benefits or desirable physiological effects. Functional attributes of many traditional foods are being discovered, while new food products are being developed with beneficial components.

Stanol and sterol esters

Stanol and sterol esters occur naturally in small quantities in many plants (fruit, vegetables, seeds, nuts, and legumes). They are available in some manufactured products in the form of yoghurts, light cream cheese, and milk (see Table 11.8).

Box 11.5 Alternatives to salt for flavouring food	
Herbs	Pepper
Spices	Vinegar
Lemon juice	Chilli
Garlic	

Table 11.8 Stanol and sterol esters included in functional food products	
1 portion =	1 yoghurt
	12 g (2.5 level teaspoons) of spread
	20 g (4 level teaspoons) of light cream cheese
	250 mL milk
Or 1 yoghurt drink/day (70 g or 100 g depending on make)	

- They decrease the absorption of both endogenous and exogenous cholesterol from the intestine. The unabsorbed cholesterol is excreted in the faeces and hence leads to a reduction in TC and LDL-C.
- 1.5–2.3 g/day stanol/sterol esters, is seen as the optimum intake.
- The average cholesterol reduction is about 10% but individual response is variable.
- The ability of a stanol/sterol ester to decrease cholesterol does not appear to be significantly different.
- The recommended intake should be eaten every day.
- They can be expensive.
- They can be taken in addition to statins as their cholesterol-lowering mechanism is different. This is not the case for ezetimibe.

Possible problems

- They may reduce the absorption of some fat-soluble vitamins, particularly beta-carotene.
- Eating increased amounts of fruit and vegetables could counter the decrease in absorption of the fat-soluble vitamins.

Dietary cholesterol

Cholesterol is a wax like substance that is essential to life as it is the primary component of animal cell membranes and a substrate for the synthesis of bile acids, steroid hormones, and vitamin D.

- Effect of dietary cholesterol on TC and LDL-C levels is modest compared with saturated fatty acids and TFAs.
- 100 mg/day of dietary cholesterol, results in a change of ~0.05 mmol/L for LDL and 0.01 mmol/L for HDL-C respectively.
- Inter-individual variation: ~15–25% of people are sensitive to dietary cholesterol (hyper-responders). The remainder have a decreased response (hypo-responders) with about a threefold difference mainly in the LDL-C response.
- 'Little evidence to support a major association between dietary cholesterol and CHD risk in the general population with the caveat that it may have a detrimental effect in hyper-responders.'[20]
- Intake of foods high in dietary cholesterol (see Table 11.9) are often associated with intake of foods high in saturated fat, so reducing saturated fat intake will in turn reduce the intake of dietary cholesterol.

Cholesterol content	Foods	Estimated cholesterol/100 g
High	Liver, offal, and products containing these	230–690 mg
	Egg yolk, and mayonnaise	1120 mg
	Fish roes	500–700 mg
	Shellfish	20–200 mg
Moderate	Fat on meat, duck, goose, and cold cuts	100 mg
	Full fat milk, cheese, butter, and cream	14–100 mg
	Pies, cakes, biscuits, and pastries	40–100 mg
Low	Fish	40–50 mg
	Very lean meats, poultry no skin	50–60 mg
	Skimmed milk, low-fat yoghurt	2–5 mg
	Bread	0–20 mg
Cholesterol free	All vegetables, vegetable oils, and nuts	0 mg
	Fruit including avocado and olives	0 mg
	Egg white, meringue, and sugar	0 mg

Table 11.9 Cholesterol content in foods

Vitamins and minerals

Epidemiological data suggests antioxidant vitamins have some beneficial effects. This reduction in mortality has not been replicated in controlled trials for beta-carotene, vitamin A, and vitamin E.[21] High doses of these antioxidants have also been shown to increase mortality risk.

Vitamin D

Vitamin D is a fat-soluble steroid hormone. It is produced in the skin after exposure to sunlight.

- Circulating levels are reduced in many chronic diseases and obesity.
- Observational studies show a higher incidence of CVD in people with low levels of circulating vitamin D. This may be due to confounding factors as they often have co-morbidities (are older, more frail, and more obese).
- Controlled trials of vitamin D supplementation have shown no benefit on CVD end points.
- Insufficient evidence exists to support vitamin D supplements to reduce CVD outcomes.

Coenzyme Q_{10}

- Coenzyme Q_{10} (CoQ_{10}) is produced by the human body and is necessary for cells to function.
- Circulating level of CoQ_{10} decreases with age and with chronic diseases and some prescription drugs.
- Supplementation with CoQ_{10} can increase the levels in the body but it is unclear whether this is beneficial.

- Some studies have shown a beneficial effect of CoQ_{10} at reducing side effects of statin therapy but the evidence is inconclusive.
- There is no evidence of harm.

Frequently asked questions

Is chocolate good for the heart?

- Some ingredients in chocolate, cocoa and flavonoids, have been linked to the prevention of CVD.
- Duration and quality of chocolate studies are poor and commercially available chocolate is not used.
- Commercial chocolate is high in fat and sugar and should be consumed in moderation.

Can garlic help reduce my cholesterol?

- Garlic has been shown to reduce cholesterol levels by a small amount.
- The robustness of the effect is debatable due to study quality and study duration.
- The implication for clinical practice is that garlic use is not an efficient way to decrease total serum cholesterol.
- However, it is a good replacement for salt when flavouring food.

Should I take a red yeast supplement?

- Red yeast extract is a supplement.
- It is a product of yeast grown on rice and is used a lot in Asian countries.
- It contains substances that inhibit cholesterol synthesis; one of these is monacolin K (also known as lovastatin), which inhibits HMG-CoA reductase.
- As it is marketed and sold as a dietary supplement, rather than as a medication, regulatory requirements are not strict enough to include mandatory information about the amount of the product included.

Do I need a folate supplement to help my homocysteine level?

- Raised homocysteine levels have been shown to be an independent marker of increased CVD risk and related to folate deficiencies.
- Folic acid supplementation trials have not shown any benefit in mortality outcomes.
- Vitamin B_{12}, vitamin B_6, and riboflavin are thought to affect homocysteine levels.
- The combination of the vitamins that will most effectively lower homocysteine levels has yet to be discovered.
- Supplements should not be recommended with a sole aim of reducing homocysteine levels but patients should be encouraged to get adequate vitamins from a cardioprotective diet.

Do I need to take cod liver oil?

- There is no substantial evidence to show the benefits of taking cod liver oil for either joint mobility or cholesterol-lowering effects.

How many eggs can I eat a week?

- As foods rich in dietary cholesterol (such as eggs and products that include egg, like mayonnaise), liver and prawns have little effect on CVD risk.
- Foods high in dietary cholesterol are often associated with intake of foods high in saturated fat. Reducing saturated fat intake and replacing with unsaturated fat can help reduce cardiovascular risk.
- The equivalent of one egg a day, with the occasional consumption of prawns or offal, all cooked in a healthy way is harmless.

Is coffee bad for the heart?

- The evidence remains unclear for the effect of coffee on CVD, probably due to how coffee is prepared.
- A lipid-rich fraction from boiled coffee may increase serum cholesterol concentrations. When the boiled coffee is filtered, the lipid-rich factor is retained in the filter paper and the effect on cholesterol is reduced substantially.
- Although there is no clear pattern, heavy coffee drinking should not be encouraged.

Is heating oil during cooking harmful?

- Heating any type of unsaturated oil at very high temperatures can result in an unfavourable change in the oil composition. Temperatures in home cooking should not be a concern provided the oil is used only once.

Dietary factors and medication interactions

Statins and grapefruit juice

Grapefruit juice can increase the bioavailability of some statins and alter pharmacokinetic and pharmacodynamic parameters.[22] The resulting increased potency may lead to an increased risk of side effects. Therefore, it is advisable to recommend avoidance of grapefruit juice during statin therapy.

Warfarin

The following factors can affect the international normalized ratio (INR) level:
- Weight gain or loss
- Change in bowel habit
- Acute illness
- Vomiting
- Smoking cessation
- Certain medications
- Diet:
  - Liver or vegetables such as Brussel sprouts, kale, spinach, chard, broccoli, and parsley are high in vitamin K and may reduce the anticoagulant effect of warfarin
  - Cranberry and grapefruit juice also increase the effect of warfarin

- Heavy alcohol intake can affect warfarin in both ways depending if the heavy drinking is acute or chronic
- Herbal and food supplements: St John's wort and glucosamine should be avoided.

Patients may receive conflicting advice from different professionals. For example, to increase fruit and vegetable intake to follow a healthier diet but due to their vitamin K level they may also be advised to restrict their intake to prevent changes in the INR. Therefore patients should be advised to try and keep their diet consistent and to make any dietary changes gradually in conjunction with close INR monitoring.

Strategies to improve dietary patterns

- Give advice and set goals through discussion and negotiation rather than in a didactic fashion. This should help to encourage a longer-term adherence.
- Make goals 'SMART' (specific, measurable, achievable, realistic, and time-specific).
- Monitor progress towards reaching goals, manage lapses and problems, and develop a contingency plan to prevent relapse.
- Brainstorm with your patients about practical advice and strategies to overcome the many different challenges that they may encounter whilst changing their dietary pattern:
  - Cooking tips
  - Shopping guidelines
  - Nutritional label reading
  - Eating out—at restaurants and family's and friends' houses
  - Cost implications—strategies on how to keep the cost down
  - Portion sizes and suitable proportions of food groups to ensure the diet remains balanced
  - Seasonal variation
- Provide support network information:
  - Support groups
  - Family and friends networks—provide ways to ensure family and friends are aware and brought on board to provide support and not create difficult situations
  - Websites and smartphone apps—ensure these are sourced from recognized and regulated institutions.

Example of how to change an unhealthy dietary pattern to a cardioprotective diet using simple changes to each meal

The changes in Table 11.10 will result in a diet low in saturated fat, and higher in unsaturated fat, fibre, fruit, vegetables, wholegrains, and low-GI foods. It also benefits from oily fish intake and reduced alcohol intake.

Dietary interventions to modify biomedical factors

Table 11.11 shows how cardiovascular risk factors can be modified with dietary changes.

	Reported diet	Cardioprotective suggestions
Breakfast	Cornflakes with whole milk Or Cheese and white bread Or Croissant with jam Coffee/tea with sugar	Porridge with low-fat milk and berries Or Unsweetened muesli with low-fat yoghurt Or Wholegrain toast with USFA spread (made from an unsaturated fatty acid) Coffee/tea no sugar
Mid-morning	Latte coffee with biscuits	Americano coffee with low-fat milk and fruit
Lunch	Sandwich containing: 2 slices of white bread Butter Cheese/salami/chicken and mayonnaise Tomato/cucumber	Sandwich containing: 2 slices of wholegrain bread USFA spread (made from an unsaturated fatty acid) Chicken/salmon, tuna/roasted vegetables Tomato/cucumber
	Salted crisps (1 packet 40 g)	Unsalted nuts (1 packet 40 g)
Mid-afternoon	Glass of fizzy soda, e.g. coke	Diet drink or fizzy water with fruit
Dinner	3 glasses red wine (150 mL each)	2 glasses red wine (125 mL each)
	Spaghetti bolognaise: White spaghetti (200 g) Minced beef/pork (fat not strained off) Sauce (tomatoes, onions, celery, mushrooms) (200 g)	Spaghetti bolognaise: Wholegrain spaghetti (100 g) Lean minced beef (replace half with lentils) Strain any fat off, add carrots, celery, mushrooms and any other vegetable
	Green salad drizzled with olive oil and balsamic vinegar	Green salad, with 1/2 an avocado, pumpkin seeds, drizzled with olive oil and balsamic vinegar
	Fruit salad with Greek yoghurt	Fruit salad with low fat natural yoghurt
Snacks	Chocolate/salted nuts	Popcorn (homemade with limited flavouring)

Table 11.10 Dietary changes to enhance cardioprotection

Weight

Obesity and cardiovascular disease risk

Obesity has become a global epidemic over the last three decades with an estimated 500 million adults being classed as obese. Overweight and obesity are associated with increased all-cause mortality. There is a J-shaped relation between BMI and the risk of death.

Central obesity

Central obesity affects lifespan due to its association with metabolic, cardiovascular, and cancer events. The distribution of fat, especially visceral fat and its relationship with

Table 11.11 Dietary changes to modify biomedical risk factors	
Biomedical factor modification	Dietary intervention[a]
Blood lipids: To reduce LDL-C	Decrease saturated fatty acids and TFAs Choose PUFA, MUFA, and soluble fibre Consider the use of stanol/sterol esters Advise weight loss in the overweight and the obese (see 'Weight' section in this chapter)
To increase HDL-C	Increase physical activity (see Chapter 12) Advise weight loss in the overweight and the obese Improve glycaemic control in diabetics Moderate alcohol consumption Advise smoking cessation
To reduce TGs	Increase physical activity Advise weight loss in the overweight and obese Improved glycaemic control Reduced alcohol consumption Reduced sugar consumption replace with soluble fibre Increase oily fish consumption/supplementation
To reduce BP	Reduce salt intake Reduce alcohol intake Increase potassium and calcium intake from fruits and vegetables Advise weight loss in the overweight and obese Increase physical activity
To reduce obesity (see 'Weight' section in this chapter)	Reduce total calorie intake Increase physical activity Set realistic weight loss target (10% in 6 months)
Manage diabetes and impaired glucose tolerance	Refer to a dietitian if glycaemic control is poor (hyper- or hypoglycaemic) Ensure regular intake of low GI foods Follow dietary recommendations for CVD management Advise weight loss in the overweight and obese

[a] All information on how to implement these interventions can be found in earlier sections of this chapter.

CVD, is independent of total body fat. It is important to measure *waist circumference* or *waist to hip ratio* in order to estimate the cardiovascular risk associated with increased abdominal obesity. Central obesity is a key driver of the metabolic syndrome which is a clustering of cardiovascular and metabolic abnormalities and hence a predictor of diabetes and CVD (see Box 11.6).

Causes of obesity

Obesity occurs when energy intake from food and drink exceeds energy expenditure through the body's metabolism and physical activity over a prolonged duration. Many complex behavioural and societal factors combine to the development of obesity. The Foresight report presents an 'obesity systems map' (see Fig. 11.1) with energy balance

Box 11.6 Abnormalities associated with obesity and central obesity

A cluster of the following substantially increases the risk of CVD:

- Insulin resistance
- Hyper-insulinaemia
- Glucose intolerance
- Type 2 diabetes
- Poor lipid profile (raised TGs; raised small-dense LDL-C, low HDL-C)
- Hypertension
- Endothelial dysfunction
- Impaired fibrinolysis and increased susceptibility to thrombosis
- Low chronic inflammation state
- Osteoarthritis
- Gout
- Sleep apnoea
- Breathlessness
- Gall bladder disease
- Cancers (colon, kidney, prostrate, breast, and endometrial)
- Infertility
- Increased anaesthetic risk.

at the centre identifying over 100 variables that either directly or indirectly may contribute to influencing energy balance. These variables have been divided into the following seven themes:

- Biology: an individual's starting point—the influence of genetics and ill health.
- Physical activity environment: the influence of the environment on an individual's activity behaviour, for example, a decision to cycle to work may be influenced by road safety, air pollution, or provision of a cycle shelter and showers.
- Physical activity: the type, frequency, and intensity of activities an individual carries out.
- Societal influences: the impact of society, for example, the influence of the media, education, peer pressure, or culture.
- Individual psychology: for example, a person's individual psychological drive for particular foods and consumption patterns, or physical activity patterns or preferences.
- Food environment: the influence of the food environment on an individual's food choices, for example, a decision to eat more fruit and vegetables may be influenced by the availability and quality of fruit and vegetables near home.
- Food consumption: the quality, quantity, and frequency (snacking patterns) of an individual's diet.

Foresight

Obesity System Map

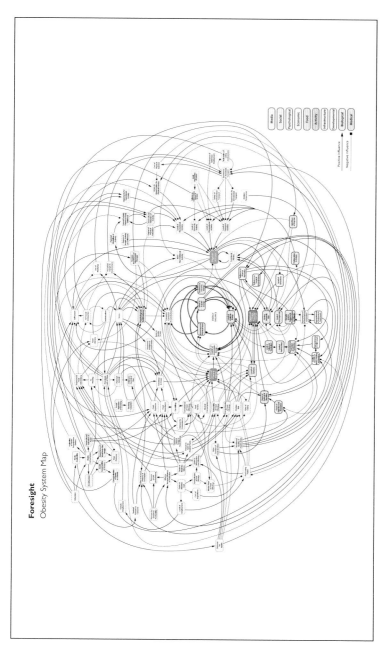

Figure 11.1 Foresight: obesity system map.

Obesity paradox

There is some evidence to show that those with excess body weight have a better outcome in patients with CVD, including heart failure.[23] The AHEAD study showed improved CVD risk factors profile but no benefit in reduced mortality.[4]

Possible explanations

- Selection bias—excess body weight can cause dyspnoea/peripheral oedema for reasons not related to heart failure, thus leading to an early diagnosis of heart failure at a stage when myocardial impairment is not yet severe.
- Good early management of the heart failure—this could also explain why obese patients with heart failure are managed more effectively, and enjoy better prognosis.
- Only 'healthy' obese patients with no co-morbidities may be surviving long enough to develop heart failure.
- Potential confounders such as smoking, unrecognized systemic illness, or unintentional weight loss may potentially account for paradoxical results.
- Chronic heart failure is a catabolic state, and the development of wasting, characterized by loss of muscle, bone, and fat, is a marker of more severe disease. Obese patients may tolerate the metabolic stress better than lean individuals.
- Altered cytokine and neuroendocrine profiles of obese patients play a role in modulating heart failure progression.
- Obese patients with co-morbidities may need to lose more weight to gain mortality benefits.

Losing a proportion of total body weight is associated with health benefits. The required proportions of weight loss to achieve different benefits vary. See below:

- Metabolic benefits: 5% weight loss
- Ventilatory, reproductive benefits: 10% weight loss
- Cardiovascular risk, anxiety, and depression, perceived health status benefits: 15% weight loss
- Eating behaviour benefits: 20% weight loss
- Activities of daily living/quality of life benefits: 25% weight loss
- Body image dysphoria benefits: 30% weight loss.

Measuring obesity and central obesity

Anthropometric measures

Anthropometric measurements provide predictions of body composition. This includes body mass, fat stores, and body water. There are a number of different measures that are available for use. The accuracy, ease of use, time to complete, and cost of each measurement varies.

Normal parameters have been set for many of the different measures (see Tables 11.12–11.14).

Table 11.12 WHO BMI recommendations		
White European population (kg/m²)	Asian population (kg/m²)	Description
<18.5	<18.5	Underweight
18.5–24.9	18.5–23	Increasing but acceptable risk
25–29.9	23–27.5	Increased risk
≥30	>27.5	High risk

Body mass index

This is an index of 'weight for height'. It is commonly used to classify underweight, overweight, and obesity in adults. This WHO classification is primarily based on the association between BMI and mortality:

$$BMI = weight(kg) / \left(height\left(m^2\right)\right)$$

The use of calculated BMI should be used with caution in the following:
- Distorted fluid balance
- High proportion of muscle mass
- Problematic height measurement (spine curvature, loss of height in elderly)
- Enforced immobility.

To measure height
- Measure without shoes, with the heels together and with the so-called Frankfurt plane of the head in a horizontal position.
- Ask the individual to breathe in deeply and reach up to a maximum height with the legs stretched and the feet flat on the ground. The height should be taken whilst the individual is looking straight ahead.
- Some weighing scales have the height measure attached.

Table 11.13 International Diabetes Federation guidance on waist circumference	
European	Men >91 cm (37 inches) Women ≥80 cm (31.5 inches)
South Asian	Men >90 cm (35 inches) Women ≥80 cm (31.5 inches)
Chinese	Men >90 cm (35 inches) Women ≥80 cm (31.5 inches)
Japanese	Men >90 cm (35 inches) Women ≥80 cm (31.5 inches)
Ethnic south and Central America	Use South Asian data until more specific ones are available
Sub-Saharan African	Use European data until more specific ones are available
Eastern Mediterranean, Middle East and Arab populations	Use European data until more specific ones are available

Table 11.14 Ideal waist:hip ratio and percentage body fat

	Men	Women
WHR	<1.0	<0.85
% fat	18–25%	25–31%

To measure weight

- Measure the subject whilst they are wearing light clothes. Ensure the removal of keys, phones, wallets, etc. from their pockets.
- Both feet should be placed firmly on the centre of the scales.
- The scales should be calibrated every year.

Waist circumference and waist:hip ratio

Waist circumference (WC) and waist:hip ratio (WHR) are both measures of abdominal obesity and are the best anthropometric predictors of cardiovascular risk. A 1 cm increase in WC is associated with a 2% increase in risk of future CVD and a 0.01 increase in WHR is associated with a 5% increase in risk.

To measure waist

- Sit in front of the individual (see Fig. 11.2).
- Ensure the individual is standing straight with both feet together (supporting themselves on a piece of furniture if they cannot balance) looking straight ahead.
- Measure next to the skin or over one piece of light clothing.

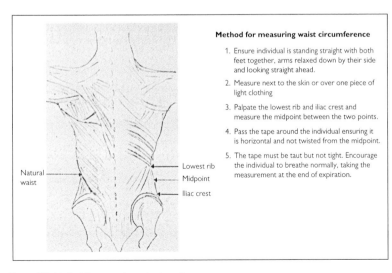

Method for measuring waist circumference

1. Ensure individual is standing straight with both feet together, arms relaxed down by their side and looking straight ahead.

2. Measure next to the skin or over one piece of light clothing

3. Palpate the lowest rib and iliac crest and measure the midpoint between the two points.

4. Pass the tape around the individual ensuring it is horizontal and not twisted from the midpoint.

5. The tape must be taut but not tight. Encourage the individual to breathe normally, taking the measurement at the end of expiration.

Natural waist —
Lowest rib —
Midpoint —
Iliac crest —

Figure 11.2 Method for measuring waist circumference.

- Measure midway between the lower rib margin and the iliac crest (see Fig. 11.2).
- Mark the level of the lowest rib margin.
- Palpate the iliac crest in the mid-axillary line and mark it.
- Pass the tape horizontally around the subject's circumference midway between the lowest rib margin and the iliac crest
- The tape should be taut but not tight. Ensure individual is relaxed and breathing normally. Take measurement on expiration.

To measure hips
- Measure at the widest point around the hips and buttocks.

$$\text{WHR} = \frac{\text{Waist in inches/cm}}{\text{Hip measurement in inches/cm}}$$

Using a visual tool to explain BMI to patients can be beneficial.
To use the BMI chart, take a straight line across from your height (without shoes) and a line up from your weight. Put a mark where the two lines meet (see Fig. 11.3).

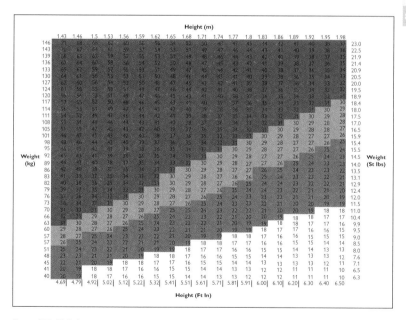

Figure 11.3 BMI chart.

Bioelectrical impedance analysis

Bioelectrical impedance analysis (BIA) is based on the principle that lean tissue is highly conductive to electrical current whereas fat is more resistant. Measurement of the changes in voltages when a current is passed through electrodes results in a measurement of total body water. Total body water can be used to estimate fat-free body mass and, by difference with body weight, body fat.

Disadvantages: it is dependent on the individual's hydration levels and does not allow for differences in body geometry.

Recent technological improvements have made BIA a more reliable and therefore more acceptable way of measuring body composition. Nevertheless it is not a 'gold standard' or reference method.

The principle of energy balance

An understanding of energy balance is indispensable for long-term weight management. If the energy you take in from your food and drink equals that of the energy you use up each day (metabolic rate and physical activity) your weight will remain stable. Altering this balance will lead to either weight gain or weight loss (see Fig. 11.4 and Box 11.7).

The imbalance only needs to be small for weight to be gained or lost. Having only 100 extra calories each day can add up to 4.5 kg (10 pounds) of weight gain in 1 year. This could be the difference between drinking a cappuccino or a latte; or changing from 100 g full fat to half fat cheese each day.

Having an energy deficit of 500–600 calories per day will usually result in about 0.5 kg (1 pound) weight loss each week. This deficit in energy balance will result in weight loss regardless of the individual's starting weight, or the type of diet consumed. Weight loss will be the result of reducing food intake and increasing physical activity.

Research has shown that long-term maintenance of weight loss has much less to do with the type of diet than the perseverance of the participants.

Characteristics of individuals who are able to maintain weight loss

- Make long-term changes to their lifestyle, not just their diet
- Monitor their progress (weight, waist, check food records, and physical activity levels)
- Set realistic goals
- Become used to eating less
- Develop healthy eating habits
- Become physically active
- Eat breakfast and plan their meals throughout the day.

Obtaining information on energy intake and dietary habits

It is well known that obese people tend to underestimate their dietary intake. Whist this confounds analysis of dietary intake, it does not invalidate valuable information on dietary habits (qualitative rather than quantitative). Particular areas of discussion with obese patients should cover the following:

- Meal patterns (regular meals and/or snacks)
- Food and drink preferences

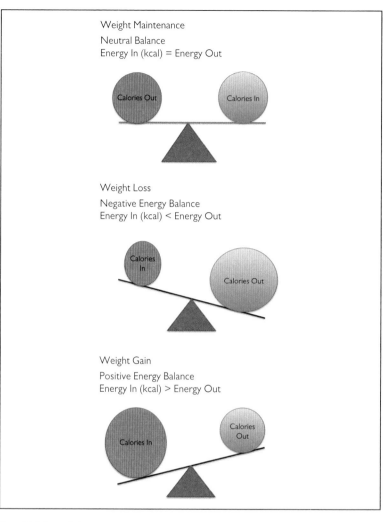

Figure 11.4 Energy balance.

- Food preparation—who is responsible for shopping and cooking?
- Work facilities—canteen, kitchen, necessity of eating outside the facilities
- Facilities at home
- Interest in food and drink
- Weekend/days off—how do eating habits differ?

> **Box 11.7 Key message for maintenance or weight changes**
>
> Energy in = energy out → weight stable.
> Energy in greater than energy out → weight gain.
> Energy in less than energy out → weight loss.

- Explore possibilities of binge, night, or emotional eating
- Portion sizes—using photographs or models can be helpful
- Alcohol intake
- Reasons for eating (hunger, boredom, comfort, stress, tiredness, and social)
- Eating outside the home or takeaways.

Energy requirements

A person's estimated energy requirements to maintain body weight can be calculated using the 'Henry formula' (see Box 11.8).[24] For this calculation the following information is required:

- Weight (kg)
- Gender
- Age
- Activity level of the individual.

The level of activity corresponds to the actual activity that the individual performs *in addition* to the normal daily exertion involved in getting up, washing, going to work, attending meals, and so on:

> **Box 11.8 Henry formula (kcal/day)**
>
> **Men**
> 18–30 years: $16.0W + 545$
> 30–60 years: $14.2W + 593$
> 60+ years: $13.5W + 514$
>
> **Women**
> 18–30 years: $13.1W + 558$
> 30–60 years: $9.74W + 694$
> 60+ years: $10.1W + 569$
>
> **Physical activity levels**
> Inactive women = BMR × 1.5
> Inactive men = BMR × 1.6
> Moderately active women = BMR × 1.6
> Moderately active men = BMR × 1.8
> Highly active women = BMR × 1.8
> Highly active men = BMR × 2.1
>
> Where BMR = basal metabolic rate and W = weight in kg.
>
> Henry CJK (2005). Basal metabolic rate studies in humans: measurement and development of new equations, *Public Health Nutrition*, 8, 7a, 1133–1152, reproduced with permission.

- Light activity: 2 hours/day active on feet
- Moderate activity: 6 hours a day active on feet
- Heavy activity: reserved for a very heavy labouring and serious athletes in training.

It is assumed that at least light activity will be encouraged for everybody. If this amount of additional exertion is not possible for medical or other reasons, then the energy requirement should be reduced by 15%.

Energy deficit for weight loss

Evidence supports a 500–600 kcal daily deficit for a 1 kg reduction in weight per week. This achieved by a combination of calorie restriction and increase in physical activity using a variety of strategies.

Pharmacological support for obesity

The one main drug option for the long-term management of obesity is orlistat. Sibutramine and rimonabant have been withdrawn due to cardiovascular and neuropsychiatric side effects.

Orlistat works in conjunction with lifestyle interventions to achieve a 5–10% weight loss, as recommended to improve cardiovascular risk profile and the risk of diabetes.

What is orlistat and what can it achieve?

- Lipase inhibitor that generates malabsorption of 30% of dietary fat
- 5–10% weight loss in 50–60% of patients and maintained for 4 years in RCTs
- Outcome is better when lifestyle support is provided
- Reduces LDL-C, diabetes incidence, and BP
- To be avoided in those with chronic diarrhoea
- Individuals taking orlistat should follow a low-fat diet as high-fat foods may cause diarrhoea.

Surgery for weight loss

Criteria for bariatric surgery

- BMI at least 40 kg/m^2
- BMI at least 35 kg/m^2 with significant co-morbidities.

Types of surgery

- Adjustable silastic gastric banding
- Gastric bypass
- Sleeve gastrectomy
- Gastric balloon.

Benefits of bariatric surgery

- Maintained weight loss—most of the weight loss occurs during the first 2 years after surgery. Weight regain may recur although it will still be significantly lower than the original weight (40–65% of preoperative weight after 5 years; 16.7% after 10 years).[25,26]

- Higher survival in patients who have undergone bariatric surgery when compared to matched severely obese, non-operated controls (SOS study)
- Improvement in cardiovascular risk factors
- Remission of chronic disease (hypertension, hyperlipidaemia, and diabetes)
- Reduced incidence of diabetes
- 33% reduced risk of total cardiovascular events and 53% reduced risk of fatal cardiovascular events.

Professional intervention

A multidisciplinary team (physician/surgeon, dietitian/nutritionist, clinical psychologist, and nurse) is essential for this type of obesity treatment. Morbidly obese people have a high anaesthetic risk of developing respiratory problems and can require intensive care unit support. Assessment must ensure the risk of the surgery does not outweigh the outcome. As well as the normal/common problems associated with surgery, these patients may also have nutritional, emotional, and psychiatric problems.

Setting targets for weight loss

Rationale for weight loss

It is essential to try and establish why an individual wants to lose weight as their level of motivation will influence their degree of success. The following questions may help identify how motivated a person is.

- Why do you want to lose weight?
  - For health/appearance/emotional reasons?
- Have you tried to lose weight before?
  - What was successful or unsuccessful?
- What support networks do you have in place?
  - Who can support you or who will not be supportive?
- How willing are you to address your physical activity levels?
  - (See also Chapter 12.)
- What are the costs and benefit of weight loss?
  - Does what you have to give up or do to achieve the weight loss goal outweigh the benefits of weight loss?
- What are the potential barriers to implementing the necessary changes?
  - Work patterns/time/family pressures.
- Are you ready and willing to make the necessary changes?
  - Have the barriers to weight loss been explored? Have strategies to avoid relapse been identified?
  - What is their stage of change? (See also Chapter 8.)

Assessing stage of change and motivation

It is important to identify an individual's motivation to lose weight and readiness to change their eating and activity behaviours. Changing behaviours and maintaining changes is key to the successful treatment of obesity. Further information on behaviour change strategies can be found in Chapter 8.

Weight

Target weights

Many people have an 'ideal weight' in their mind when they set out to lose weight, which are often unrealistic as targets and regarding the time frame. Research has shown that an individual who is overweight or obese can vastly improve their health by losing as little as 10% of their present body weight (see Box 11.9).

Practical strategies for weight loss

Self-monitoring

Keep food, exercise, and mood diaries as these can:

- form part of continuous assessment and intervention
- help to identify patterns
- increase awareness
- record progress
- highlight new problems
- serve as a motivational indicator.

Monitoring itself can reduce intake. Higher rates of weight loss are associated with more accurate self-monitoring.

Setting behavioural goals and making a change plan

Goals should be SMART (see Box 11.10).

Rewards

Set small, realistic, easily achievable goals regularly rather than long-term distal ones. This is motivational because it leads to 'quick wins'. Ensure that these short-term goals are relevant to the overall objective.

Box 11.9 Benefits of 10 kg weight loss in a 100 kg subject

- Mortality: 20–25% decrease in premature mortality
- BP:
  - 10 mmHg decrease in SBP
  - 20 mmHg decrease in DBP
- Lipids:
  - 10% decrease in TC
  - 15% decrease in LDL-C
  - 8% increase in HDL-C
  - 30% decrease in TGs
- Diabetes:
  - 50% decrease in risk of developing type 2 diabetes
  - 30–50% decrease in elevated blood glucose
  - 15% decrease in HbA1c.

Box 11.10 Setting SMART goals

- Specific: do you know exactly what you need to do?
- Measurable: how will you know when you've achieved your goal?
- Achievable: is this a goal you can realistically achieve?
- Relevant to the goal of treatment: is this goal helping you move towards the larger goal you are trying to achieve?
- Time-specific: when are you going to achieve this goal?

Managing internal and external triggers

Reduce exposure, modify response, and use cognitive behavioural therapy strategies. See Table 11.15.

Problem-solving

- What is the problem situation? For example, a birthday party.
- What is my plan? (Generate different solutions, assess pros and cons of each solution):
  - Healthy eating for the rest of the day
  - Identify how many unhealthy foods can be eaten and then move away from food area
  - Practice in advance what to say when offered inappropriate food
  - Speak to person having party to ensure there are some healthy options available
- Did you manage to stick to the plan?
  - Identify success or failure and learn from the process

Enlisting social support

- Social barriers (e.g. lack of social support) are a major contributor to poor adherence

Table 11.15 Possible internal and external triggers to eating

Internal triggers	External triggers
Boredom/loneliness	Lack of time
Anger/frustration/tension/anxiety	Routine/lack of routine
Feeling high/low	Forgot to do shopping/shopping when hunger
Stress	
Disappointment/resentment	Social situations/cooking for others
Unassertiveness (too shy to ask for alternative or say no)	No suitable foods
	Others tempting you/passing shops
Negative thoughts	Eating alone
Cravings	Smell of food
Physiological triggers (hunger, thirst, changes in metabolic rate, weight loss)	

- Other people can be helpful or unhelpful
- Identify family members, friends, and situations that will be helpful (be specific!)
- Encourage a problem-solving approach to getting the right type of support
- Communicating the plan to others is important as they may not understand how important the change is and how they can help!

Weight cycling

Weight maintenance and prevention of weight cycling is an enormous challenge for people who have succeeded in the short term in a weight-loss programme as weight is often gradually regained.

People who achieve the most in the long term are those who:

- make modest changes to their diet
- lose weight gradually
- monitor themselves
- continue with a healthy diet
- take regular exercise.[27]

How to reduce calorie intake

Swapping foods

By replacing high calorie foods with lower calorie foods. For example:

- Vanilla ice cream for a fruit sorbet: 139 kcal saved
- Caesar salad or salad with light dressing: 140 kcal saved
- ½ cup fried rice to ½ cup steamed rice: 53 kcal saved
- Café latte to cappuccino: 80 kcal saved
- 100 g full-fat cream cheese to low-fat cream cheese: 144 kcal saved.

This method is often effective for people who have routine in their lives because it is relatively easy to identify which foods or drinks can be swapped to reduce the calorie intake enough to promote weight loss.

Reducing total intake

In simply reducing the overall intake of foods normally eaten, take care if the overall dietary pattern is not healthy. Although reducing the intake will aid weight loss, maintenance may be more difficult.

For example:

- 2 slices of toast rather than 3
- 3 tablespoons of rice rather than 4
- 85 g (3 oz) of meat (one deck of playing cards) rather than 170 g (6 oz) (two decks of playing cards)
- 1 teaspoon of mayonnaise rather than 1 dessertspoon.

This approach often works well for people who have little or no routine in their lives and are very busy. But focus must also be given to ways of improving the diet to bring it in line with the cardioprotective recommendations.

Changing the proportion of food groups in the diet

This method may help people to reduce their calorie intake by changing the proportion of food groups within the diet. As shown in the plate models (see Fig. 11.5), it encourages the reduction of protein and carbohydrate foods and replaces them with fruit and vegetables so the total volume remains the same, but the healthy balance is improved.

The tip with this method is to add the vegetables to the plate first followed by starchy food and then finally to add the protein food. This idea needs to be applied to all meals. Ask your patient to draw their plate next to the meal described in their food diary.

High-protein/low-carbohydrate diets

These diets will induce weight loss initially from glycogen and water losses. Protein is highly satiating and therefore less is consumed; however, conclusive evidence for its

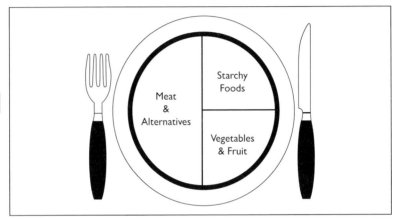

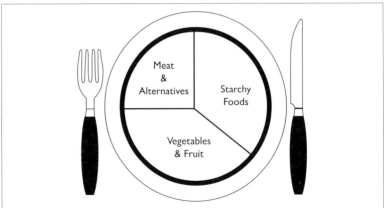

Figure 11.5 Plate models.
Image reproduced with permission from Dietetic Department. Imperial NHS Trust.

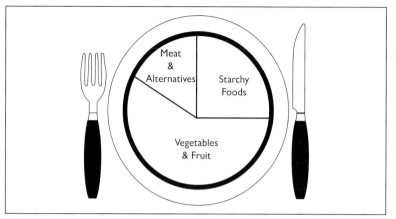

Figure 11.5 Continued

Table 11.16 Comparing products			
	Per 100 g		
	Low	Moderate	High
Total fat/sugar	<3 g	2–20 g	>20 g
Saturated fat	<1.5 g	1.5–5 g	>5 g

effectiveness is lacking and long-term data regarding its effect on CVD risk factors are limited.

Hidden calories

Awareness of hidden calories in food and drinks is essential. Product marketing may make the food appear healthy, but a closer look at the content often reveals high levels of fat or sugar (e.g. some muesli bars with yoghurt, 98% fat-free biscuits/cakes, and 'light' butter). Therefore it is essential to be able to interpret nutritional information on food product labels. Using the per 100 g/100 mL column facilitates comparison of products (see Table 11.16).

References

1. Estruch R, Martinez-Gonzalez MA, Corella D, *et al.* Effects of a Mediterranean-style diet on cardiovascular risk factors: a randomized trial. *Ann Intern Med* 2006; 145:1–11.

2. Slimani N, Deharveng G, Charrondiere RU, *et al.* Structure of the standardized computerized 24-h diet recall interview used as reference method in the 22 centers participating in the EPIC project. European Prospective Investigation into Cancer and Nutrition. *Compt. Methods Programs Biomed* 1999;58:251–266.

3. Kromhout D, Keys A, Aravanis C, *et al.* Food consumption patterns in the 1960s in seven countries. *Am J Clin Nutr* 1989; 49:889–94.

4. AHEAD study. http://www.ncbi.nlm.nih.gov/pubmed/21836103 *Diabetes Care* 2011 Oct; 34(10):2152–7. doi: 10.2337/dc11-0874. Epub Aug 2011.

5. Jenkins DJ, Kendall CW, Marchie A, *et al*. Direct comparison of a dietary portfolio of cholesterol-lowering foods with a statin in hypercholesterolemic participants. *Am J Clin Nutr* 2005; 81:380–7.

6. Jenkins DJ, Kendall CW, Faulkner DA, *et al*. Long-term effects of a plant-based dietary portfolio of cholesterol-lowering foods on blood pressure. *Eur J Clin Nutr* 2008; 62:781–8.

7. Albert CM, Hennekens CH, O'Donnell CJ, et al. Fish consumption and risk of sudden cardiac death. *JAMA* 1998; 279:23–28.

8. Hu FB, Bronner L, Willett WC, *et al*. Fish and omega-3 fatty acid intake and risk of coronary heart disease in women. *JAMA* 2002; 287:1815–1821.

9. Burr ML, Fehily AM, Gilbert JF, *et al*. Effects of changes in fat, fish, and fibre intakes on death and myocardial reinfarction: diet and reinfarction trial (DART). *Lancet* 1989; 2(8666):757–61.

10. Gruppo Italiano per lo Studio della Sopravvivenza nell'Infarto. Dietary supplementation with n-3 polyunsaturated fatty acids and vitamin E after myocardial infarction: results of the GISSI-Prevenzione trial. *Lancet* 1999; 354(9177):447–55.

11. Gissi-HF Investigators, Tavazzi L, Maggioni AP, *et al*. Effect of n-3 polyunsaturated fatty acids in patients with chronic heart failure (the GISSI-HF trial): a randomised, double-blind, placebo-controlled trial. *Lancet* 2008; 372(9645):1223–30.

12. Mente A, De Koning L, Shannon HS, *et al*. (2009). A systematic review of the evidence supporting a causal link between dietary factors and coronary heart disease. *Arch Intern Med* 2009; 169:659–69.

13. Threapleton DE, Greenwood DC, Evans CE, *et al*. Dietary fibre intake and risk of cardiovascular disease: systematic review and meta-analysis. *BMJ* 2013; 347:f6879.

14. Fung TT, Malik V, Rexrode KM, *et al*. Sweetened beverage consumption and risk of coronary heart disease in women. *Am J Clin Nutr* 2009; 89(4):1037–42.

15. de Koning L, Malik VS, Kellogg MD, *et al*. Sweetened beverage consumption, incident coronary heart disease, and biomarkers of risk in men. *Circulation* 2012; 125(14):1735–41.

16. Sabate J, Oda K, Ros E. Nut consumption and blood lipid levels: a pooled analysis of 25 intervention trials. *Arch Intern Med* 2010; 170:821–7.

17. Mattes RD, Dreher ML. Nuts and healthy body weight maintenance mechanisms. *Asia Pac J Clin Nutr* 2010; 19:137–41.

18. Anderson JW, Johnstone BM, Cook-Newell ME. Meta-analysis of the effects of soy protein intake on serum lipids. *N Engl J Med* 1995; 333:276–282.

19. Rimm EB, Klatsky A, Grobbee D, *et al*. Review of moderate alcohol consumption and reduced risk of coronary heart disease: is the effect due to beer, wine, or spirits. *BMJ* 1996; 312:731–6.

20. Djousse L, Gaziano JM. Dietary cholesterol and coronary artery disease: a systematic review. *Curr Atheroscler Rep* 2009; 11:418–22.

21. Bjelakovic G, Nikolova D, Gluud LL, *et al*. Antioxidant supplements for prevention of mortality in healthy participants and patients with various diseases. *Cochrane Database Syst Rev* 2008; 2:CD007176.

22. Dahan A, Altman H. Food-drug interaction: grapefruit juice augments drug bioavailability – mechanism, extent and relevance. *Eur J Clin Nutr* 2004; 58(1):1–9.

23. Arena R, Lavie CJ. The obesity paradox and outcome in heart failure: is excess bodyweight truly protective? *Future Cardiol* 2010; 6:1–6.

24. Henry CJ. Basal metabolic rate studies in humans: measurement and development of new equations. *Public Health Nutr* 2005; 8:1133–52.

25. Kral JG. Overview of surgical techniques for treating obesity. *Am J Clin Nutr* 1992; 55:552S–5S.

26. Sjöström L. Surgical intervention as a strategy for treatment of obesity. *Endocrine* 2000; 13:213–30.

27. Skender ML, Goodrick GK, Del Junco DJ, *et al*. Comparison of 2-year weight loss trends in behavioral treatments of obesity: diet, exercise, and combination interventions. *J Am Diet Assoc* 1996; 96:342–6.

Chapter 12

Helping people to become more physically active

Key messages

- There is a cause–effect relationship linking a sedentary lifestyle to cardiovascular risk.
- Helping people to become more physically active is essential to effective primary and secondary cardiovascular prevention.
- Several possible types of interventions based on different approaches are available.
- The choice of intervention should be based on both individual and community perspectives and should be based on a compromise between available scientific evidence and cost-effectiveness considerations.

Summary

- This chapter describes multilevel initiatives to support individuals and families in increasing their physical activity levels.

The imperative

- A sedentary lifestyle is an important risk factor for CVD.
- Less than 50% of people in Europe indulge in regular aerobic physical activity.
- Physical activity interventions can be implemented at population/community and family/individual levels—these interventions are cost-effective.

Consider the support you provide as a health professional to your patients to help them to become more physically active in the context of the political and social environment and other initiatives that facilitate adoption of your advice.

What are the barriers?

- Convincing stakeholders that physical activity interventions are beneficial:
  - Why?
  - Because confirming that the effects of physical activity interventions can be sustained in the long term is challenging.

- Accurate measurement of physical activity is problematic:
  - Why?
  - Because using self-reported measures (e.g. questionnaires) may be subject to bias, and objective measures (e.g. accelerometers), may underestimate actual levels of physical activity undertaken.

Possible barriers to implementation of a public health plan for physical activity

- Public health plan for physical activity development
- Appropriately trained staff
- Financial support
- Access to physical activity content expertise
- Political will and support from agency
- Community partners and leaders in physical activity
- Access to state and local data on physical activity.

Decisions to implement physical activity interventions should be based on evidence-based criteria (see Box 12.1), if possible derived from scientific evidence specific to the population being considered as the object of the intervention.

Interventions to promote physical activity

Interventions used to promote physical activity can be classified into three categories, according to the approach used (see Box 12.2).

Providing information

- This approach aims to motivate people not only to modify their behaviour, but also to maintain that modified behaviour over time.
- It aims to provide knowledge about the benefits of physical activity, increase awareness of opportunities for increasing physical activity, explain methods for overcoming barriers and negative attitudes about physical activity, and increase participation in community-based activities.

Box 12.1 Criteria for decision-making about physical activity promotion

- Evidence-based effectiveness.
- Evidence-based cost.
- Evidence-based benefits.
- Distribution of costs and benefits.
- Fairness.
- Political support.

Providing information
Changing knowledge and attitudes about the benefits of and opportunities for physical activity within a community.

Behavioural and social
Teaching people the behavioural management skills necessary both for successful adoption and maintenance of behaviour change and for creating social environments that facilitate and enhance behavioural change.

Environmental and policy
Structuring physical and organizational environments to provide safe, attractive, and convenient places for physical activity.

Examples of how this approach is used are shown in the following sections.

Point-of-decision prompts

For example, signs placed by lifts may motivate people to use nearby stairs instead (see Fig. 12.1).

- Signs can remind people of opportunities at hand to be more active and gain benefits to their health.
- Prompts should be tailored to the target population in order to increase effectiveness of the intervention.
- The advice on the sign should be easy to follow, for example, the stairway should be easy to find and well lit, maintained, and safe.

Evidence

- Point-of-decision prompts have been found to be cost-effective with a median of £0.05/MET-hour/day/person, because they are inexpensive and reach a large population (where 1 MET (metabolic equivalent of task) = 1 kcal/kg/hour).
- However, their effectiveness is limited to meeting only 0.2% of guideline-recommended levels of physical activity and so should be used together with other approaches to increasing physical activity.

Community campaigns

- Involve the whole community.
- Are highly visible and broad-based.
- Can be directed at the population via various media, for example, the Internet, television, radio, newspapers, direct mailings, billboards, advertisements in transit outlets, and trailers in cinemas.
- May include social support using self-help groups, risk factor screening, counselling, and educational initiatives in a variety of settings, including worksites, schools, and community events.
- May include environmental or policy changes such as the creation of walking trails.

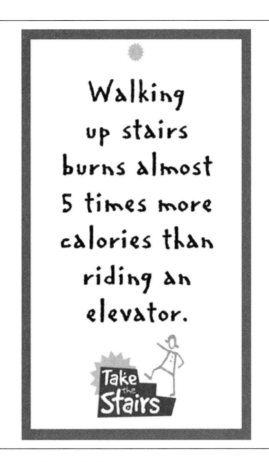

Figure 12.1 An example of a point-of-decision prompt.

This approach has the added benefit of building social networks, actively involving community members in local government and civic organizations, and so increasing social capital and resulting in a greater sense of cohesion and collective self-efficacy.

Examples of campaigns from around the world

The *Lazy Town* (http://www.lazytown.com) TV series is an example from Iceland, which encourages and inspires children in a fun and creative way to adopt a healthy diet and daily physical activity. *Lazy Town* has been aired in over 128 countries worldwide and in 500 million homes (see Fig. 12.2).

In the United States, the web-based 'Let's Move!' campaign (http://www.letsmove.gov) aims to fight childhood obesity using a five-step approach (see Fig. 12.3) which has different tracks for parents, children, and schools. It includes:

- revamping labelling of nutritional products by the Department of Agriculture

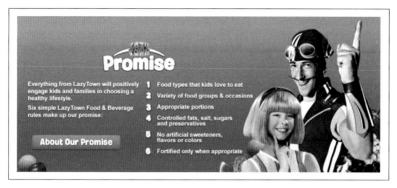

Figure 12.2 Lazy Town initiative.

- improving the nutritional standards of the National School Lunch Program
- increasing children's opportunities to be physically active
- improving community access to high-quality foods.

An example from Let's Move! of how to get started to 'make physical activity a part of your family's routine' is reported in Box 12.3.

The United Kingdom Department of Health has implemented the 'Change4Life' public health campaign (see Fig. 12.4), a web-based initiative which uses three key messages: 'eat well', 'move more' and 'live longer'. The Change4Life website (http://www.nhs.uk/Change4Life/Pages/change-for-life.aspx) advocates improving the quality of both eating and physical activity habits, and at the same time provides links to find activities in one's local area and to social networks (Change4Life is on Twitter and Facebook).

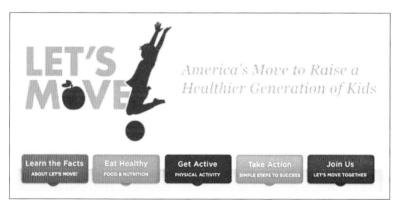

Figure 12.3 Let's Move! initiative.

Box 12.3 'Ideas to get started' from Let's Move!

- Play tag, swim, toss a ball, jump rope, hula-hoop, dance to music, or even play a dancing video game. It doesn't have to be sports—just get your family moving!
- Walk the dog, go for a jog, go on a bike ride, take the stairs, or head to the park and let kids run around for a while.
- Celebrate special occasions—like birthdays or anniversaries—with something active, such as a hike, a volleyball or soccer game, or playing Frisbee at the park.
- Get the whole family involved in household chores like cleaning, vacuuming, and yard work.
- Walk instead of drive whenever you can. If you have to drive, find a spot at the far end of the parking lot and walk to where you're going.
- Park farther away and count with your children the number of steps from the car to your destination. Write it down and see if you can park even farther away on your next stop.
- Train as a family for a charity walk or run.

Evidence

In spite of the social resonance of such initiatives, their cost-effectiveness and the gain provided in recommended physical activity levels are not yet clearly established (see Fig. 12.5).

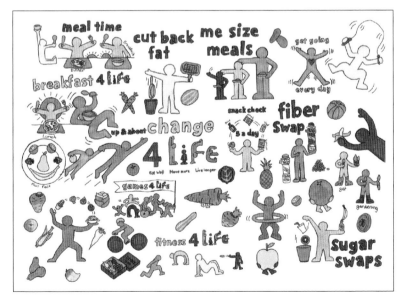

Figure 12.4 Change4Life initiative in the United Kingdom.

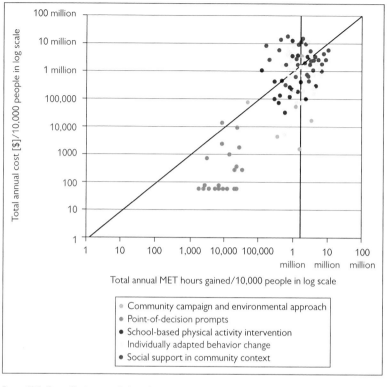

Figure 12.5 Cost-effectiveness of physical activity promotion initiatives.

Classroom-based health education

Health education classes that provide information and skills related to decision-making are usually multicomponent, with the curriculum typically addressing physical activity, nutrition, smoking, and CVD. Health education classes, taught in infant, primary, and secondary schools, are designed to effect behaviour change through personal and behavioural factors that provide students with the skills they need for rational decision-making.

Rather than changes in activity, this kind of intervention is likely to increase general health knowledge, exercise-related knowledge, and self-efficacy about exercise.

Behavioural and social approach

- These approaches focus on teaching widely applicable management skills and by structuring the social environment to provide support for people trying to initiate or maintain behaviour change.

- Adding new (or additional) physical exercise classes.
- Lengthening existing physical exercise classes.
- Increasing moderate to vigorous physical activity of students during physical exercise class without necessarily lengthening class time (e.g. changing the activities taught or modifying the rules of the game so that students are more active).

- Interventions often involve individual or group behavioural counselling and typically include the friends or family members that constitute an individual's social environment.
- Skills focus on recognizing cues and opportunities for physical activity, ways to manage high-risk situations, and ways to maintain behaviour and prevent relapse.
- Interventions also involve making changes in the home, family, school, and work environments.

Examples of these approaches are shown in the following sections.

School-based intervention

Curricula and policies to increase the amount of time students spend in moderate or vigorous activity at school are modified as shown in Box 12.4.

- The aim is to set long-term behavioural patterns during the transition to adulthood using didactic and behavioural methods.
- These initiatives do not have to be offered by physical exercise or wellness departments in college and university settings, but they do include supervised exercise in the class setting.
- Students can apply these lessons in practical sessions in which they engage in supervised physical activity, develop goals and activity plans, and write term papers based on their experiences.
- Students are also encouraged to support each other using phone calls etc. They also agree to behavioural contracts for an agreed-on amount of physical activity.
- In infant and primary schools, as an alternative to interventions aimed at increasing the amount of time students spend in physical activity, teachers can hold classes that specifically emphasize decreasing the amount of time spent watching television and playing video games.
- Students are taught techniques and strategies to self-monitor progression towards goals to limit television viewing and video gaming.

Evidence

School-based physical activity interventions targeted at children and adolescents are relatively cost-effective (median £0.28/MET-hour/day/person) when no additional school staff's labour costs are required. These interventions generate a median of 0.48 MET-hours, a quantity equivalent to 16% of the guideline-recommended physical activity for youth (Fig. 12.6).

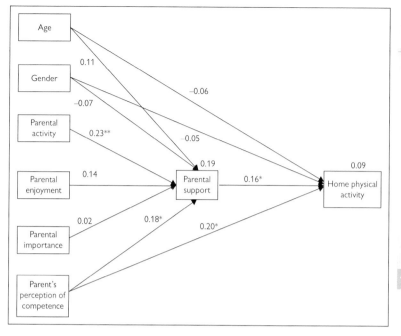

Figure 12.6 Increasing physical activity in school children.

Family-based social support

- These approaches focus on increasing support within the family for behaviour change.
- The family is considered the most important setting for shaping children's physical activity.
- Parents provide a role model for children, for example, by participating in sport with their children, or accompanying children to sports training and events, providing money and clothing for activity, and encouraging physical activity and the physical environment within the home (Fig. 12.7).
- A supportive social environment increases maintenance of behaviour change.
- Interventions may be targeted to families with children or to spouses or partners without children.
- Programmes typically include joint or separate educational sessions on health, goal-setting, problem-solving, or family behavioural management and will often incorporate some physical activities.
- Interventions in this category targeted to children and their families are often implemented as part of a larger strategy that includes other school-based

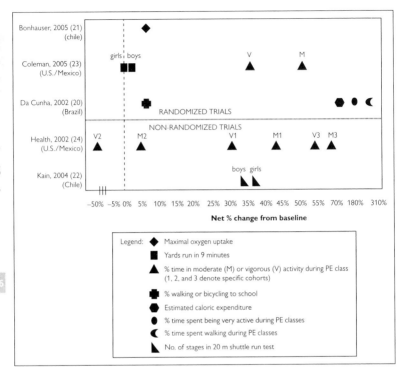

Figure 12.7 Parental support for children to increase physical activity levels.

interventions, such as school-based physical exercise or classroom-based health education.

● In this setting, the family component is often conceptualized as an adjunct home curriculum to the school activities, involving take-home packets, reward systems, and family record keeping.

Community-based social support

● These approaches focus on building, strengthening, and maintaining social networks that provide supportive relationships for behaviour change either by creating new social networks or working within pre-existing networks in a social setting outside the family, such as the workplace.

● Interventions typically involve making a 'contract' with others to achieve specified levels of physical activity, or setting up walking or other groups to provide companionship and support while being physically active.

● There is strong evidence that social support interventions in community settings are effective in increasing levels of physical activity, as measured by an increase in the percentage of people engaging in physical activity, energy expenditure, or other measure of physical activity.

Evidence

- Programmes that are more costly per MET-hour gained include high-intensity individually adapted behaviour change (see later) and social support programmes, with a median of £0.55 and £0.77/MET-hour/day/person, respectively.
- These programmes are less cost-effective primarily because they involve intensive face-to-face counselling or interaction.
- Although more intensive interventions generate larger effect sizes (0.53 and 0.65 MET-hours/day, respectively, or about 35% and 43% of the guideline-recommended physical activity for adults), the increase in effect size does not match the increase in costs compared to low-cost interventions.

Individually adapted health behaviour change

- These programmes are tailored to the individual's readiness for change (see Chapter 8), specific interests, and preferences.
- They teach specific behavioural skills that enable participants to incorporate physical activity into daily routines. Behaviours may be planned (e.g. a daily scheduled walk) or unplanned (e.g. taking the stairs when the opportunity arises).
- Many or most of these interventions use constructs from one or more established health behaviour change models such as social cognitive theory, the health belief model, or the transtheoretical model of change (see Chapter 8).
- The behavioural approaches used in individually adapted health behaviour change programmes are shown in Box 12.5.
- All of these interventions are delivered to people either in group settings or by mail, telephone, or directed media.
- Individually adapted health behaviour change programmes require careful planning and coordination, well-trained staff members, and resources sufficient to carry out the programme as planned.
- Inadequate resources and lack of professionally trained staff members may affect how completely and appropriately interventions are implemented and evaluated.

Box 12.5 Behavioural approaches for individually adapted health behaviour change

- Setting goals for physical activity and self-monitoring of progress toward goals.
- Building social support for new behavioural patterns.
- Behavioural reinforcement through self-reward and positive self-talk.
- Structured problem-solving geared to maintenance of the behaviour change.
- Prevention of relapse into sedentary behaviours.

Evidence

There is strong evidence that individually adapted health behaviour change programmes are effective in increasing levels of physical activity, even if with the cost-effectiveness limitations highlighted earlier.

Environmental and policy approach

- These approaches are designed to provide environmental opportunities, support, and cues to help people develop healthier behaviours.

Table 12.1 The Neighborhood Environment Walkability Scale

Subscale	Sample Items
Residential density	How common are detached single-family residences in your immediate neighborhood? How common are apartments or condors 1–3 stories in your immediate neighborhood?
Land use mix-diversity	About how long would it take to get from your home to the *nearest* businesses or facilities if you walked to them? Convinience/small grocery store • Post office • Video store • Non-fast food restaurant
Land use mix-access	I can do most of my shopping at local stores. Parking is difficult in local shopping areas.
Street connectivity	The streets I my neighborhood do not have many, or any, cul-de-sacs. The distance between intersections in my neighborhood is usually short.
Walking/cycling facilities	The sidewalks in my neighborhood are well maintained. There is a grass/dirt strip that separates the streets from sidewalks in my neighborhood.
Aesthetics	There are many attractive natural sights in my neighborhood (such as landscaping, views). There are attractive buildings/homes in my neighborhood.
Pedestrain/automobile traffic safety	The speed of traffic on most nearby streets is usually slow (30 mph or less). There are crosswalks and pedestrain signals to hepl walkers cross busy streets in my neighborhood.
Crime safety	There is a high crime rate in my neighborhood. My neighborhood streets are well lit at night.

Note: The complete Neighborhood Environment Walkability Scale (NEWS) and scoring procedures are available at http://www.drjamessallis.sdsu.edu/NEWS.pdf and http://www.drjamessallis.sdsu.edu/NEWSscoring.pdf, respectively.

- Correlational studies have shown that physical activity levels are associated with factors such as the availability of exercise equipment in the home and the proximity and density of places for physical activity within neighbourhoods.
- Other neighbourhood and environmental characteristics such as safety lighting, weather, and air pollution also affect physical activity levels, regardless of individual motivation and knowledge.
- Specific scales have been developed to evaluate how amenable a neighbourhood is to promoting physical activity, such as the Neighborhood Environment Walkability Scale (see Table 12.1).
- Areas with a high density of family households in close proximity to shops, services, bus, tram, and train stops, pavements, cycle paths, low-cost recreational facilities, and reasonable safety from crime are associated with meeting the physical activity guidelines, either by walking alone or from overall physical activity (see Fig. 12.8).

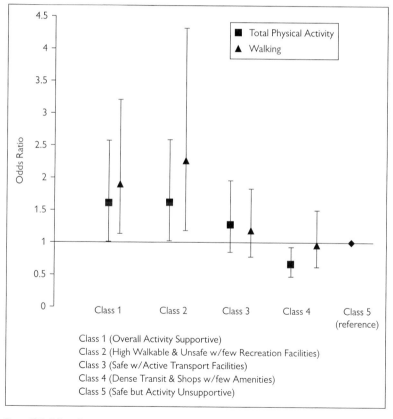

Figure 12.8 Safety of environment.

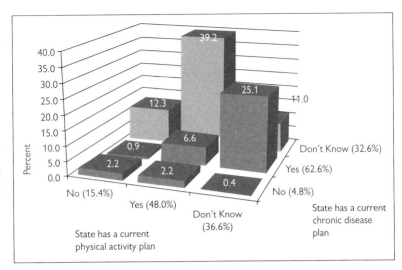

Figure 12.9 State plans for physical activity.

- To have a population effect, environmental and policy interventions are not directed to individuals but rather to physical and organizational structures, and are usually implemented and evaluated over a longer period of time than more individually oriented interventions.
- Interventions are conducted by conventional health professionals, but they also involve many sectors that have not previously been associated with public health, such as community agencies and organizations, legislators, and the mass media.
- The goal is to increase physical activity through changing social networks, organizational norms and policies, the physical environment, resources and facilities, and laws.
- Of note, several physical activity practitioners have been found to believe either that state public health plans for physical activity already exist, although the contrary often is true, or to know nothing about the existence of such plans (see Fig. 12.9). This highlights once more the need for an adequate dissemination of physical activity-related information.

Creation of or enhanced access to places for physical activity

Worksites, coalitions, agencies, and communities can create or provide access to places and facilities where people can be physically active (see Box 12.6).

Evidence

- This type of intervention is effective in increasing physical activity in diverse settings and populations, provided appropriate attention is paid to adapting the intervention to the target population.

- Provision of access to weight and aerobic fitness equipment in fitness or community centres.
- The creation of walking trails.
- Provision of access to nearby fitness or leisure centres.

- One potential barrier is that building new facilities is time- and resource-consuming.
- Creation of enhanced access requires careful planning and coordination.
- Success is greatly enhanced by community buy-in, which can take a great deal of time and effort to achieve.

Key reading

Jørgensen T, Capewell S, Prescott E, *et al.* Population-level changes to promote cardiovascular health. *Eur J Prev Cardiol* 2013; 20(3):409–21.

Longmuir PE, Brothers JA, de Ferranti SD, *et al.* Promotion of physical activity for children and adults with congenital heart disease: a scientific statement from the American Heart Association. *Circulation* 2013; 127(21):2147–59.

Pate RR, Davis MG, Robinson TN, *et al.* Promoting physical activity in children and youth: a leadership role for schools: a scientific statement from the American Heart Association Council on Nutrition, Physical Activity, and Metabolism (Physical Activity Committee) in collaboration with the Councils on Cardiovascular Disease in the Young and Cardiovascular Nursing. *Circulation* 2006; 114(11):1214–24.

Warren JM, Ekelund U, Besson H, *et al.* Assessment of physical activity – a review of methodologies with reference to epidemiological research: a report of the exercise physiology section of the European Association of Cardiovascular Prevention and Rehabilitation. *Eur J Cardiovasc Prev Rehabil* 2010; 17(2):127–39.

Wu S, Cohen D, Shi Y, *et al.* Economic analysis of physical activity interventions. *Am J Prev Med* 2011; 40(2):149–58.

Chapter 13

Managing blood pressure

Key messages

- High BP is a major public health problem; 30–45% of European adults are hypertensive, and similar figures apply to all developed societies.
- There is a continuous relationship between increasing BP and CVD risk.
- The impact on risk is modulated by other risk factors and by the presence of end-organ damage so total risk should be assessed.
- Ambulatory BP monitoring is valuable for diagnosis, risk stratification, and assessment of the effectiveness of treatment.
- Effective treatment through lifestyle and appropriate drug treatment unequivocally reduces CVD mortality and morbidity.
- Effective BP control is more important than the agent chosen.
- Combination drug therapy is often required.
- Older people are more prone to side effects such as postural hypotension.

Summary

- Raised BP is one of the biggest global public health challenges. It relates to salt intake and overweight but is multifactorial in origin and also frequently occurs in the absence of these factors. It interacts with smoking and hyperlipidaemia to greatly increase total risk.
- BP rises with age but this does not make it safe—the relationship with risk continues. Twenty-four-hour ambulatory BP monitoring is becoming a 'standard of care' to refine risk assessment and the efficacy of treatment.
- Effective BP control through lifestyle advice and judicious use of drug treatment reduces CVD risk. Thresholds for treatment and targets are defined. Management can be more challenging than in hyperlipidaemia in that a combination of several drugs is often required.

Epidemiological aspects

Relationship of blood pressure to cardiovascular and renal damage

- There is an independent continuous relationship between office BP and incidence of cardiovascular events and end-stage renal disease; this is true of all ages and ethnic groups.

- The relation with BP extends from higher levels to relatively low values of 110–115 mmHg for systolic BP (SBP) and 70–75 mmHg for diastolic BP (DBP) in individuals with no previous manifest CVD.
- SBP appears to be a better predictor of events than DBP after the age of 50.
- A continuous relationship with events is also exhibited by out-of-office BP values (ambulatory BP monitoring/home BP monitoring).

Definition and classification of hypertension

There is no change in the definition and classification of hypertension in the 2013 ESH/ESC guidelines compared to the previous 2007 guidelines (see Table 13.1).

Prevalence of hypertension

- Prevalence of hypertension in the general population in Europe is 30–45% (based on 21 publications from the last decade), increasing with age.
- Stroke mortality can be used as a surrogate of hypertension status.

Hypertension and total cardiovascular risk

Prevention of CHD should be related to quantification of total cardiovascular risk, which is summarized in Table 13.2.

For more than a decade, international guidelines for the management of hypertension have stratified cardiovascular risk in different categories based on BP levels, cardiovascular risk factors, asymptomatic organ damage, and presence of diabetes, symptomatic CVD, or chronic kidney disease.

The same approach is presented in Fig. 13.1. The factors used for risk stratification are explained in Table 13.3.

Table 13.1 Definitions and classification of office BP levels (mmHg)[a]

Category	Systolic		Diastolic
Optimal	<120	and	<80
Normal	120–129	and/or	80–84
High normal	130–139	and/or	85–89
Grade 1 hypertension	140–159	and/or	90–99
Grade 2 hypertension	160–179	and/or	100–109
Grade 3 hypertension	≥180	and/or	≥110
Isolated systolic hypertension	≥140	and	<90

[a]The blood pressure (BP) category is defined by the highest level of BP, whether systolic or diastolic. Isolated systolic hypertension should be graded 1, 2, or 3 according to systolic BP values in the ranges indicated.

G. Mancia, R. Fagard, K. Narkiewicz, 2013 ESH/ESC Guidelines for the management of arterial hypertension, *European Heart Journal*, 2013; 34(28):2159–219 by permission of Oxford University Press.

Table 13.2 Total cardiovascular risk assessment		
Recommendations	Class[a]	Level[b]
In asymptomatic subjects with hypertension but free of CVD, CKD, and diabetes, total CV risk stratification using the SCORE model is recommended as a minimal requirement.	I	B
As there is evidence that OD predicts CV death independently of SCORE, a search for OD should be considered, particularly in individuals at moderate risk.	IIa	B
It is recommended that decisions on treatment strategies depend on the initial level of total CV risk.	I	B

CKD = chronic kidney disease; CV = cardiovascular; CVD = cardiovascular disease; OD = organ damage; SCORE = Systematic COronary Risk Evaluation.

[a]Class of recommendation.

[b]Level of evidence.

G. Mancia, R. Fagard, K. Narkiewicz, 2013 ESH/ESC Guidelines for the management of arterial hypertension, *European Heart Journal*, 2013; 34(28):2159–219 by permission of Oxford University Press.

Diagnostic evaluation

The initial evaluation of a patient with hypertension should:

* confirm the diagnosis of hypertension
* rule out causes of secondary hypertension
* assess cardiovascular risk, organ damage, and concomitant clinical conditions.

Other risk factors, asymptomatic organ damage or disease	Blood Pressure (mmHg)			
	High normal SBP 130–139 or DBP 85–89	Grade 1 HT SBP 140–159 or DBP 90–99	Grade 2 HT SBP 160–179 or DBP 100–109	Grade 3 HT SBP ≥180 or DBP ≥110
No other RF		Low risk	Moderate risk	High risk
1–2 RFs	Low risk	Moderate risk	Moderate to high risk	High risk
≥3 RFs	Low to Moderate risk	Moderate to high risk	High risk	High risk
OD, CKD stage 3 or diabetes	Moderate to high risk	High risk	High risk	High to Very high risk
Symptomatic CVD, CKD stage ≥4 or diabetes with OD/RFs	Very high risk	Very high risk	Very high risk	Very high risk

BP = blood pressure; CKD = chronic kidney disease; CV = cardiovascular; CVD = cardiovascular disease; DBP = diastolic blood pressure; HT = hypertension; OD = organ damage; RF = risk factor; SBP = systolic blood pressure.

Figure 13.1 Stratification of total cardiovascular risk in categories of low, moderate, high, and very high risk according to SBP and DBP and prevalence of risk factors.

G. Mancia, R. Fagard, K. Narkiewicz, 2013 ESH/ESC Guidelines for the management of arterial hypertension, *European Heart Journal*, 2013; 34(28):2159–219 by permission of Oxford University Press.

Table 13.3 Factors—other than office BP—influencing prognosis; used for stratification of total cardiovascular risk

Risk factors

Male sex

Age (men ≥55 years; women ≥65 years)

Smoking

Dyslipidaemia

  Total cholesterol >4.9 mmol/L (190 mg/dL), and/or

  Low-density lipoprotein cholesterol >3.0 mmol/L (115 mg/dL), and/or

  High-density lipoprotein cholesterol: men <1.0 mmol/L (40 mg/dL), women <1.2 mmol/L (46 mg/dL), and/or

  Triglycerides >1.7 mmol/L (150 mg/dL)

Fasting plasma glucose 5.6–6.9 mmol/L (102–125 mg/dL)

Abnormal glucose tolerance test

Obesity [BMI ≥30 kg/m^2 (height^2)]

Abdominal obesity (waist circumference: men ≥102 cm; women ≥88 cm) (in Caucasians)

Family history of premature CVD (men aged <55 years; women aged <65 years)

Asymptomatic organ damage

Pulse pressure (in the elderly) ≥60 mmHg

Electrocardiographic LVH (Sokolow–Lyon index >3.5 mV; RaVL >1.1 mV; Cornell voltage duration product >244 mV*ms), or

Echocardiographic LVH [LVM index: men >115 g/m^2; women >95 g/m^2 (BSA)][a]

Carotid wall thickening (IMT >0.9 mm) or plaque

Carotid–femoral PWV >10 m/s

Ankle-brachial index <0.9

CKD with eGFR 30–60 mL/min/1.73 m^2 (BSA)

Microalbuminuria (30–300 mg/24 h), or albumin/creatinine ratio (30–300 mg/g; 3.4–34 mg/mmol) (preferentially on morning spot urine)

Diabetes mellitus

Fasting plasma glucose ≥7.0 mmol/L (126 mg/dL) on two repeated measurements, and/or

HbA$_{1c}$ >7% (53 mmol/mol), and/or

Post-load plasma glucose >11.0 mmol/L (198 mg/dL)

Established CV or renal disease

Cerebrovascular disease: ischaemic stroke; cerebral haemorrhage; transient ischaemic attack

(continued)

Table 13.3 Continued

Risk factors

CHD: myocardial infarction; angina; myocardial revascularization with PCI or CABG

Heart failure, including heart failure with preserved EF

Symptomatic lower extremities peripheral artery disease

CKD with eGFR <30 mL/min/1.73m² (BSA); proteinuria (>300 mg/24 h).

Advanced retinopathy: haemorrhages or exudates, papilloedema

BMI = body mass index; BP = blood pressure; BSA = body surface area; CABG = coronary artery bypass graft; CHD = coronary heart disease; CKD = chronic kidney disease; CV = cardiovascular; CVD = cardiovascular disease; EF = ejection fraction; eGFR = estimated glomerular filtration rate; HbA_{1c} = glycated haemoglobin; IMT = intima-media thickness; LVH = left ventricular hypertrophy; LVM = left ventricular mass; PCI = percutaneous coronary intervention; PWV = pulse wave velocity.

[a]Risk maximal for concentric LVH: increased LVM index with a wall thickness/radius ratio of > 0.42.

G. Mancia, R. Fagard, K. Narkiewicz, 2013 ESH/ESC Guidelines for the management of arterial hypertension, *European Heart Journal*, 2013; 34(28):2159–219 by permission of Oxford University Press.

Blood pressure measurement

- Office BP is recommended for screening and diagnosis of hypertension.
- Diagnosis of hypertension should be based on at least two BP measurements per visit and on at least two visits.
- Out-of-office BP monitoring (ambulatory BP monitoring or home BP monitoring) should be considered to confirm the diagnosis of hypertension, identify the type of hypertension, detect hypotensive episodes, and maximize prediction of cardiovascular risk.

Caution: cut-off values for the definition of hypertension differ for office and out-of-office BP (see Table 13.4).

Personal and family history

Caution: do not forget to ask about the use of drugs/substances affecting BP: oral contraceptives, liquorice, carbenoxolone, vasoconstrictive nasal drops, cocaine, amphetamines, gluco- and mineralocorticosteroids, non-steroidal anti-inflammatory drugs, erythropoietin, and ciclosporin.

Physical examination

- All patients should undergo auscultation of the carotid arteries, heart, and renal arteries.
- Height, weight, and waist circumference should be measured with the patient standing, and BMI calculated.
- Resting heart rate should be measured in all patients.
- Radiofemoral delay should be assessed as a check for coarctation of the aorta.

Table 13.4 Definitions of hypertension by office and out-of-office BP levels			
Category	Systolic BP (mmHg)		Diastolic BP (mmHg)
Office BP	≥140	and/or	≥90
Ambulatory BP			
Daytime (or awake)	≥135	and/or	≥85
Nighttime (or asleep)	≥120	and/or	≥70
24-h	≥130	and/or	≥80
Home BP	≥135	and/or	≥85

BP = blood pressure.

G. Mancia, R. Fagard, K. Narkiewicz, 2013 ESH/ESC Guidelines for the management of arterial hypertension, *European Heart Journal*, 2013; 34(28):2159–219 by permission of Oxford University Press.

Laboratory investigations

Laboratory investigations are summarized in Table 13.5.

Predictive value, availability, reproducibility, and cost-effectiveness of some markers of organ damage are presented in Table 13.6.

Treatment approach

Administration of BP-lowering drugs is supported by the following evidence:
- Reduction of risk of major clinical cardiovascular outcomes
- Regression of organ damage.

Fig. 13.2 summarizes indications for the initiation of lifestyle changes and antihypertensive drug treatment according to the level of total cardiovascular risk as in Fig. 13.1.

When to initiate antihypertensive drug treatment

Initiation of antihypertensive drug treatment is summarized in Table 13.7.

Blood pressure treatment goals

Generally, the recommended BP goals are less radical than in the previous guidelines, and are presented in Table 13.8.

Treatment strategies

Lifestyle changes

The following lifestyle changes are recommended:
- Salt restriction to 5–6 g/day
- Moderation of alcohol consumption (<20–30 g of ethanol/day in men, and <10–20 g of ethanol/day in women)
- Increased consumption of vegetables, fruits, and low-fat dairy products
- Reduction of body weight in overweight and obese individuals

Table 13.5 Laboratory investigations

Routine tests

- Haemoglobin and/or haematocrit

- Fasting plasma glucose

- Serum total cholesterol, low-density lipoprotein cholesterol, high-density lipoprotein cholesterol

- Fasting serum triglycerides

- Serum potassium and sodium

- Serum uric acid

- Serum creatinine (with estimation of GFR)

- Urine analysis: microscopic examination; urinary protein by dipstick test; test for microalbuminuria

- 12-lead ECG

Additional tests, based on history, physical examination, and findings from routine laboratory tests

- Haemoglobin A_{1c} (if fasting plasma glucose is >5.6 mmol/L (102 mg/dL) or previous diagnosis of diabetes)

- Quantitative proteinuria (if dipstick test is positive); urinary potassium and sodium concentration and their ratio

- Home and 24-h ambulatory BP monitoring

- Echocardiogram

- Holter monitoring in case of arrhythmias

- Exercise testing

- Carotid ultrasound

- Peripheral artery/abdominal ultrasound

- Pulse wave velocity

- Ankle-brachial index

- Fundoscopy

Extended evaluation (mostly domain of the specialist)

- Further search for cerebral, cardiac, renal, and vascular damage, mandatory in resistant and complicated hypertension

- Search for secondary hypertension when suggested by history, physical examination, or routine and additional tests

BP = blood pressure; ECG = electrocardiogram; GFR = glomerular filtration rate.

G. Mancia, R. Fagard, K. Narkiewicz, 2013 ESH/ESC Guidelines for the management of arterial hypertension, *European Heart Journal*, 2013; 34(28):2159–219 by permission of Oxford University Press.

Table 13.6 Predictive value, availability, reproducibility, and cost-effectiveness of some markers of organ damage

Marker	Cardiovascular predictive value	Availability	Reproducibility	Cost-effectiveness
Electrocardiography	+++	++++	++++	++++
Echocardiography, plus Doppler	++++	+++	+++	+++
Estimated glomerular filtration rate	+++	++++	++++	++++
Microalbuminuria	+++	++++	++	++++
Carotid intima–media thickness and plaque	+++	+++	+++	+++
Arterial stiffness (pulse wave velocity)	+++	++	+++	+++
Ankle–brachial index	+++	+++	+++	+++
Fundoscopy	+++	++++	++	+++
Additional measurements				
Coronary calcium score	++	+	+++	+
Endothelial dysfunction	++	+	+	+
Cerebral lacunae/white matter lesions	++	+	+++	+
Cardiac magnetic resonance	++	+	+++	++

Scores are from + to ++ + +.

G. Mancia, R. Fagard, K. Narkiewicz, 2013 ESH/ESC Guidelines for the management of arterial hypertension, *European Heart Journal*, 2013; 34(28):2159–219 by permission of Oxford University Press.

- Regular exercise (at least 30 minutes of moderate dynamic exercise on 5–7 days per week)
- Quitting smoking!

Drug treatment

Choice of antihypertensive treatment

- The main benefit of antihypertensive treatment is due to lowering of BP per se, and is largely independent of the drugs employed.
- Therefore, the five major classes of antihypertensive drugs (diuretics, beta blockers, calcium antagonists, ACEIs, and angiotensin receptor blockers (ARBs)) are all suitable for the initiation and maintenance of antihypertensive treatment, either in monotherapy or in some combination, taking into account compelling and possible contraindications (Table 13.9) and specific conditions for some drugs to be preferred (Table 13.10).

Other risk factors, asymptomatic organ damage or disease	Blood Pressure (mmHg)			
	High normal SBP 130–139 or DBP 85–89	Grade 1 HT SBP 140–159 or DBP 90–99	Grade 2 HT SBP 160–179 or DBP 100–109	Grade 3 HT SBP ≥189 or DBP ≥110
No other RF	• No BP intervention	• Lifestyle changes for several months • Then add BP drugs targeting <140/90	• Lifestyle changes for several weeks • Then add BP drugs targeting <140/90	• Lifestyle changes • Immediate BP drugs targeting <140/90
1–2 RFs	• Lifestyle changes • No BP intervention	• Lifestyle changes for several weeks • Then add BP drugs targeting <140/90	• Lifestyle changes for several weeks • Then add BP drugs targeting <140/90	• Lifestyle changes • Immediate BP drugs targeting <140/90
≥3 RFs	• Lifestyle changes • No BP intervention	• Lifestyle changes for several weeks • Then add BP drugs targeting <140/90	• Lifestyle changes • BP drugs targeting <140/90	• Lifestyle changes • Immediate BP drugs targeting <140/90
OD, CKD stage 3 or diabetes	• Lifestyle changes • No BP intervention	• Lifestyle changes • BP drugs targeting <140/90	• Lifestyle changes • BP drugs targeting <140/90	• Lifestyle changes • Immediate BP drugs targeting <140/90
Symptomatic CVD, CKD stage ≥4 or diabetes with OD/RFs	• Lifestyle changes • No BP intervention	• Lifestyle changes • BP drugs targeting <140/90	• Lifestyle changes • BP drugs targeting <140/90	• Lifestyle changes • Immediate BP drugs targeting <140/90

BP = blood pressure; CKD = chronic kidney disease; CV = cardiovascular; CVD = cardiovascular disease; DBP = diastolic blood pressure; HT = hypertension; OD = organ damage; RF = risk factor; SBP = systolic blood pressure.

Figure 13.2 Initiation of lifestyle changes and antihypertensive drug treatment.
G. Mancia, R. Fagard, K. Narkiewicz, 2013 ESH/ESC Guidelines for the management of arterial hypertension, *European Heart Journal*, 2013; 34(28):2159–219 by permission of Oxford University Press.

Monotherapy and combination therapy

- No matter which drug is employed, monotherapy can effectively reduce BP only in a limited number of hypertensive patients.
- Most patients require the combination of at least two drugs to achieve BP control. Combination therapy results in:
  - a prompt response in a larger number of patients (potentially beneficial in high-risk patients)
  - a greater probability of achieving target BP in patients with higher initial BP values
  - improved adherence.
- Mineralocorticoid receptor antagonists, amiloride, and the alpha-1-blocker doxazosin should be considered for combination treatment of resistant hypertension.

Table 13.7 Initiation of antihypertensive drug treatment

Recommendations	Class[a]	Level[b]
Prompt initiation of drug treatment is recommended in individuals with grade 2 and 3 hypertension with any level of CV risk, a few weeks after or simultaneously with initiation of lifestyle changes.	I	A
Lowering BP with drugs is also recommended when total CV risk is high because of OD, diabetes, CVD or CKD, even when hypertension is in the grade 1 range.	I	B
Initiation of antihypertensive drug treatment should also be considered in grade 1 hypertensive patients at low to moderate risk, when BP is within this range at several repeated visits or elevated by ambulatory BP criteria, and remains within this range despite a reasonable period of time with lifestyle measures.	IIa	B
In elderly hypertensive patients drug treatment is recommended when SBP is ≥160 mmHg.	I	A
Antihypertensive drug treatment may also be considered in the elderly (at least when younger than 80 years) when SBP is in the 140–159 mmHg range, provided that antihypertensive treatment is well tolerated.	IIb	C
Unless the necessary evidence is obtained it is not recommended to initiate antihypertensive drug therapy at high normal BP.	III	A
Lack of evidence does also not allow recommending to initiate antihypertensive drug therapy in young individuals with isolated elevation of brachial SBP, but these individuals should be followed closely with lifestyle recommendations.	III	A

BP = blood pressure; CKD = chronic kidney disease; CV = cardiovascular; CVD = cardiovascular disease; OD = organ damage; SBP = systolic blood pressure.

[a]Class of recommendation.

[b]Level of evidence.

G. Mancia, R. Fagard, K. Narkiewicz, 2013 ESH/ESC Guidelines for the management of arterial hypertension, *European Heart Journal*, 2013; 34(28):2159–219 by permission of Oxford University Press.

The monotherapy versus combination therapy strategies are presented in Fig. 13.3. Fig. 13.4 shows the possible combinations of classes of antihypertensive drugs. *Caution:* the combination of ACEIs and ARBs is not recommended.

Treatment of associated risk factors

Table 13.11 summarizes recommendations regarding lipid-lowering drugs, antiplatelet therapy, and treatment of hyperglycaemia in patients with hypertension.

Table 13.8 BP goals in hypertensive patients

Recommendations	Class[a]	Level[b]
A SBP goal <140 mmHg:		
a) is recommended in patients at low–moderate CV risk;	I	B
b) is recommended in patients with diabetes;	I	A
c) should be considered in patients with previous stroke or TIA;	IIa	B
d) should be considered in patients with CHD;	IIa	B
e) should be considered in patients with diabetic or non-diabetic CKD.	IIa	B
In elderly hypertensives less than 80 years old with SBP ≥160 mmHg there is solid evidence to recommend reducing SBP to between 150 and 140 mmHg.	I	A
In fit elderly patients less than 80 years old SBP values < 140 mmHg may be considered, whereas in the fragile elderly population SBP goals should be adapted to individual tolerability.	IIb	C
In individuals older than 80 years and with initial SBP ≥160 mmHg, it is recommended to reduce SBP to between 150 and 140 mmHg provided they are in good physical and mental conditions.	I	B
A DBP target of <90 mmHg is always recommended, except in patients with diabetes, in whom values <85 mmHg are recommended. It should nevertheless be considered that DBP values between 80 and 85 mmHg are safe and well tolerated.	I	A

CHD = coronary heart disease; CKD = chronic kidney disease; CV = cardiovascular; DBP = diastolic blood pressure; SBP = systolic blood pressure; TIA = transient ischaemic attack.

[a]Class of recommendation.

[b]Level of evidence.

G. Mancia, R. Fagard, K. Narkiewicz, 2013 ESH/ESC Guidelines for the management of arterial hypertension, *European Heart Journal*, 2013; 34(28):2159–219 by permission of Oxford University Press.

Follow-up

Follow-up of individuals with high normal BP or white-coat hypertension

Individuals with high normal BP or white-coat hypertension, even if untreated, should be scheduled for regular follow-up, at least annually, to measure office and out-of-office BP, to check their cardiovascular risk profile, and to reinforce recommendations on lifestyle changes.

Table 13.9 Compelling and possible contraindications to the use of anti-hypertensive drugs

Drug	Compelling	Possible
Diuretics (thiazides)	Gout	Metabolic syndrome Glucose intolerance Pregnancy Hypercalcaemia Hypokalaemia
Beta-blockers	Asthma A–V block (grade 2 or 3)	Metabolic syndrome Glucose intolerance Athletes and physically active patients Chronic obstructive pulmonary disease (except for vasodilator beta-blockers)
Calcium antagonists (dihydropyridines)		Tachyarrhythmia Heart failure
Calcium antagonists (verapamil, diltiazem)	A–V block (grade 2 or 3, trifascicular block) Severe LV dysfunction Heart failure	
ACE inhibitors	Pregnancy Angioneurotic oedema Hyperkalaemia Bilateral renal artery stenosis	Women with child bearing potential
Angiotensin receptor blockers	Pregnancy Hyperkalaemia Bilateral renal artery stenosis	Women with child bearing potential
Mineralocorticoid receptor antagonists	Acute or severe renal failure (eGFR <30 mL/min) Hyperkalaemia	

A-V = atrio-ventricular; eGFR = estimated glomerular filtration rate; LV = left ventricular.

G. Mancia, R. Fagard, K. Narkiewicz, 2013 ESH/ESC Guidelines for the management of arterial hypertension, *European Heart Journal*, 2013; 34(28):2159–219 by permission of Oxford University Press.

Follow-up of hypertensive patients

- After the initiation of antihypertensive therapy, the patients should be seen at 2- to 4-week intervals to evaluate the effect on BP, and to assess possible side effects.
- Once the BP target is reached, a visit interval of a few months is reasonable (3- to 6-month intervals).
- Risk factors and asymptomatic organ damage are recommended to be assessed at least every 2 years.

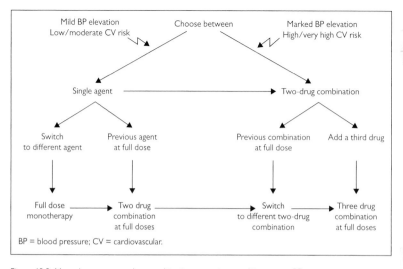

Figure 13.3 Monotherapy versus drug combination strategies to achieve target BP.

G. Mancia, R. Fagard, K. Narkiewicz, 2013 ESH/ESC Guidelines for the management of arterial hypertension, *European Heart Journal*, 2013; 34(28):2159–219 by permission of Oxford University Press.

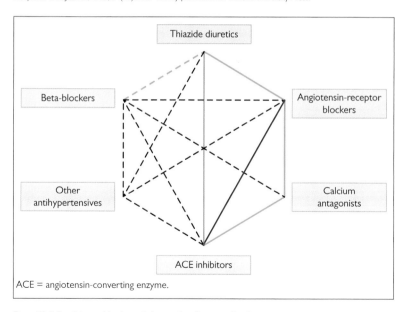

Figure 13.4 Possible combinations of classes of antihypertensive drugs.

G. Mancia, R. Fagard, K. Narkiewicz, 2013 ESH/ESC Guidelines for the management of arterial hypertension, *European Heart Journal*, 2013; 34(28):2159–219 by permission of Oxford University Press.

Table 13.10 Drugs to be preferred in specific conditions

Condition	Drug
Asymptomatic organ damage	
LVH	ACE inhibitor, calcium antagonist, ARB
Asymptomatic atherosclerosis	Calcium antagonist, ACE inhibitor
Microalbuminuria	ACE inhibitor, ARB
Renal dysfunction	ACE inhibitor, ARB
Clinical CV event	
Previous stroke	Any agent effectively lowering BP
Previous myocardial infarction	BB, ACE inhibitor, ARB
Angina pectoris	BB, calcium antagonist
Heart failure	Diuretic, BB, ACE inhibitor, ARB, mineralocorticoid receptor antagonist
Aortic aneurysm	BB
Atrial fibrillation, prevention	Consider ARB, ACE inhibitor, BB or mineralocorticoid receptor antagonist
Atrial fibrillation, ventricular rate control	BB, non-dihydropyridine calcium antagonist
ESRD/proteinuria	ACE inhibitor, ARB
Peripheral artery disease	ACE inhibitor, calcium antagonist
Other	
ISH (elderly)	Diuretic, calcium antagonist
Metabolic syndrome	ACE inhibitor, ARB, calcium antagonist
Diabetes mellitus	ACE inhibitor, ARB
Pregnancy	Methyldopa, BB, calcium antagonist
Blacks	Diuretic, calcium antagonist

ACE = angiotensin-converting enzyme; ARB = angiotensin receptor blocker; BB = beta-blocker; BP = blood pressure; CV = cardiovascular; ESRD = end-stage renal disease; ISH = isolated systolic hypertension; LVH = left ventricular hypertrophy.

G. Mancia, R. Fagard, K. Narkiewicz, 2013 ESH/ESC Guidelines for the management of arterial hypertension, *European Heart Journal*, 2013; 34(28):2159–219 by permission of Oxford University Press.

Table 13.11 Treatment of risk factors associated with hypertension.

Recommendations	Class[a]	Level[b]
It is recommended to use statin therapy in hypertensive patients at moderate to high CV risk, targeting a low-density lipoprotein cholesterol value <3.0 mmol/L (115 mg/dL).	I	A
When overt CHD is present, it is recommended to administer statin therapy to achieve low-density lipoprotein cholesterol levels <1.8 mmol/L (70 mg/dL).	I	A
Antiplatelet therapy, in particular low-dose aspirin, is recommended in hypertensive patients with previous CV events.	I	A
Aspirin should also be considered in hypertensive patients with reduced renal function or a high CV risk, provided that BP is well controlled.	IIa	B
Aspirin is not recommended for CV prevention in low-moderate risk hypertensive patients, in whom absolute benefit and harm are equivalent.	III	A
In hypertensive patients with diabetes, a HbA$_{1c}$ target of <7.0% is recommended with antidiabetic treatment.	I	B
In more fragile elderly patients with a longer diabetes duration, more comorbidities and at high risk, treatment to a HbA$_{1c}$ target of <7.5–8.0% should be considered.	IIa	C

BP = blood pressure; CHD = coronary heart disease; CV = cardiovascular; HbA$_{1c}$ = glycated haemoglobin.

[a]Class of recommendation.

[b]Level of evidence.

G. Mancia, R. Fagard, K. Narkiewicz, 2013 ESH/ESC Guidelines for the management of arterial hypertension, *European Heart Journal*, 2013; 34(28):2159–219 by permission of Oxford University Press.

Key reading

Mancia G, Fagard R, Narkiewicz K, *et al*. 2013 ESH/ESC guidelines for the management of arterial hypertension: the Task Force for the Management of Arterial Hypertension of the European Society of Hypertension (ESH) and of the European Society of Cardiology (ESC). *Eur Heart J* 2013; 34:2159–219.

Chapter 14

Managing blood lipids

Key messages

- Blood lipids should be evaluated in the context of total risk.
- Targets for the different categories of total CVD risk are defined in this chapter.
- Higher-risk people gain most from treatment.
- Check fasting lipids if possible and consider secondary causes of hyperlipidaemia, especially hypothyroidism.
- Explain to the patient the evidence base for therapy, that drugs control but do not cure hyperlipidaemia, and that treatment is lifelong.
- Know that high TGs can be very sensitive to lifestyle change.

Summary

- Hypercholesterolaemia, particularly raised LDL-C, relates to CVD in a graded manner and the relationship is causal. There is unequivocal evidence that treatment of hyperlipidaemia reduces CVD events.
- European guidelines retain a targeted approach—the higher the risk, the more intense the therapeutic advice. Current American guidance is for high-dose statin therapy for all very high-risk subjects.
- High TGs and low HDL-C signal increase risk but trials do not support target values.
- High TGs are associated with central obesity, hypertension, low HDL-C, and raised blood sugar. They may respond to weight control and alcohol reduction.
- Statins may increase blood sugar levels but the benefit associated with LDL lowering outweighs the adverse effect of this.

Which lipids should be measured?

Dyslipidaemias, that is, disturbed blood lipids are among the most important risk factors for CVD. Four lipid parameters are usually determined:

- TC
- LDL-C
- HDL-C
- TGs.

If possible, blood sampling should be made after 12 hours of fasting (this is in fact requested only for measuring TGs but the level is needed for calculation of LDL-C). LDL-C can be measured directly but is usually calculated using Friedwald's formula unless TGs are 4.5 mmol/L (~400 mg/dL) or higher:

$$LDL - C = TC - HDL - C - (0.45 \times TG) \text{ in mmol/L or}$$

$$LDL - C = TC - HDL - C - (0.2 \times TG) \text{ in mg/dL}$$

TC, HDL-C, and TGs are always measured directly. For some other lipid variables, particularly those calculated such as non-HDL-C and apolipoprotein B/apolipoprotein A ratio, it is still not established whether they should be used as treatment goals.

TC is used for the estimation of total CVD risk but is not enough for the characterization of dyslipidaemia before the beginning of treatment and is not recommended as target for treatment.

Intervention targets

There are no 'normal' levels of TC or LDL-C. LDL-C is the main target for dyslipidaemia treatment and the target levels should be achieved according to the total CVD risk (see Table 14.1).

There are no established treatment targets for TG or for HDL-C which is an independent risk factor for CVD. However, the risk is increased according to the following factors (see Box 14.1).

Management of hypercholesterolaemia

TC and LDL-C can be increased either because of inborn genetic errors of lipid metabolism or lifestyle or combination of both (see Box 14.2). However, secondary elevation of TC and LDL-C also exists.

Refer to Fig. 14.1 for a management algorithm if you suspect secondary hypercholesterolaemia.

Table 14.1 LDL-C target levels depending upon total CVD risk

Total CVD risk	LDL-C target level
Very high	<1.8 mmol/L (~70 mg/dL) or ≥50% LDL-C reduction
High	<2.5 mmol/L (~100 mg/dL)
Moderate and low	<3.0 mmol/L (~115 mg/dL)

Box 14.1 Levels of TGs and HDL-C associated with increased risk

- TG (fasting): >1.7 mmol/L (~150 mg/dL)
- HDL-C:
  - Men: <1.0 mmol/L (~40 mg/dL)
  - Women: <1.2 mmol/L (~45 mg/dL).

Box 14.2 Possible causes of secondary hypercholesterolaemia

- Hypothyroidism
- Diabetes mellitus
- Nephrotic syndrome
- Cushing syndrome
- Liver diseases
- Some medications: corticosteroids, diuretics and antihypertensives (e.g. furosemide, hydrochlorothiazide, chlorthalidone, and beta-blockers), immunosuppressives (e.g. ciclosporin), and highly active antiretroviral drugs
- Pregnancy
- Anorexia nervosa
- Lupus erythematosus
- Some malignant diseases (e.g. multiple myeloma).

Check for underlying disease

↓

Treat the disease

↓

When the disease is under control, check TC and LDL-C

↓

If not at target, consider dyslipidaemia treatment

Figure 14.1 Suspicion of hypercholesterolaemia.

Table 14.2 Intervention strategies as a function of total CVD risk and LDL-C level

Total CV risk	LDL-C levels				
	< 70 mg/dL <1.8 mmol/L	70 to < 100 mg/dL 1.8 to < 2.5 mmol/L	100 to < 155 mg/dL 2.5 to < 4.0 mmol/L	155 to < 190 mg/dL 4.0 to < 4.9 mmol/L	> 190 mg/dL > 4.9 mmol/L
Low risk	No lipid intervention	No lipid intervention	Lifestyle intervention	Lifestyle intervention	Lifestyle intervention, consider drug if uncontrolled
Moderate risk	Lifestyle intervention	Lifestyle intervention	Lifestyle intervention, consider drug if uncontrolled	Lifestyle intervention, consider drug if uncontrolled	Lifestyle intervention, consider drug if uncontrolled
High risk	Lifestyle intervention consider drug*	Lifestyle intervention consider drug*	Lifestyle intervention and immediate drug intervention	Lifestyle intervention and immediate drug intervention	Lifestyle intervention and immediate drug intervention
Very high risk	Lifestyle intervention consider drug*	Lifestyle intervention and immediate drug intervention	Lifestyle intervention and immediate drug intervention	Lifestyle intervention and immediate drug intervention	Lifestyle intervention and immediate drug intervention

* In patients with MI, statin therapy should be considered irrespective of LDL-C level.

If no secondary hypercholesterolaemia exists or elevated LDL-C persists despite adequate control of the underlying disease, intervention strategies should be applied depending upon the risk level (see Table 14.2 and Box 14.3).

If with lifestyles intervention LDL-C target values cannot be achieved, it should be continued but additional pharmacological treatment is necessary (see Box 14.4).

Box 14.3 Lifestyle interventions to lower TC and LDL-C

- Reduce dietary saturated fats and cholesterol intake (eat more fish, soy products, fruits, and vegetables and much less red meat and high-fat dairy products)
- Reduce dietary TFA intake (contained in many baking shortenings, spreads, etc.)
- Eat foods enriched with phytosterols or take phytosterol supplements
- Increase dietary fibre intake
- Reduce excessive body weight
- Take red yeast supplements.

Box 14.4 Pharmacological treatment of elevated LDL-C

- Statins are the drugs of choice for treatment of hypercholesterolaemia.
- Statins should be titrated up to the highest recommended dose or highest tolerable dose to reach the target LDL-C level.
- In case of intolerance of one statin, another statin in low dose should be introduced instead.
- In case of intolerance of all the statins, a bile acid sequestrant is recommended.
- If LDL-C target level is not achieved with a statin alone, a cholesterol absorption inhibitor can be added to decrease LDL-C further.
- If LDL-C target is not achieved with a combination of a statin and a cholesterol absorption inhibitor, additional bile acid sequestrant or nicotinic acid can be added in combination to decrease LDL-C further.

When the target LDL-C level is achieved, the same treatment should be continued permanently.

All patients with familial hypercholesterolaemia (FH) (see Table 14.4) should be considered as high-risk patients and treated with statins to achieve the appropriate LDL-C target level.

Table 14.3 Diagnostic criteria for the clinical diagnosis of heterozygous familial hypercholesterolaemia according to MEDPED and WHO

Family history	First-degree relative known with premature CAD and/or first-degree relative with LDL–C > 95th centile	1
	First-degree relative with tendon xantomata and/or children < 18 with LDL-C > 95th centile	2
Clinical history	Patient has premature CAD*	2
	Patient has premature cerebral/peripheral vascular disease	1
Physical examination	Tendon xantomata	6
	Arcus cornealis below the age of 45 years	4
LDL-C	> 8.5 mmol/L (more than ~330 mg/dL)	8
	6.5–8.4 mmol/L (~250–329 mg/dL)	5
	5.0–6.4 mmol/L (~190–249 mg/dL)	3
	4.0–4.9 mmol/L (~155–189 mg/dL)	1
Definite FH		Score > 8
Probable FH		Score 6–8
Possible FH		Score 3–5
No diagnosis		Score < 3

*Premature CAD = male before 55, women before 60 years of age.

Box 14.5 Some medicines that may increase the risk of adverse effects when used concomitantly with a statin

- Azole antifungals (ketoconazole, itraconazole, fluconazole, voriconazole)
- Macrolides (erythromycin, clarithromycin, azithromycin, telithromycin)
- Some antidepressants (nefazodone, venlafaxine, fluvoxamine, fluoxetine, sertraline)
- Midazolam
- Calcium antagonists (mibefradil, diltiazem, verapamil)
- Amiodarone
- Digoxin
- Gemfibrozil
- Ciclosporin, tacrolimus
- Tamoxifen
- HIV protease inhibitors (ritonavir, indinavir, amprenavir, nelfinavir, saquinavir, lopinavir)
- Warfarin, phenindione
- Corticosteroids
- Grapefruit juice.

Since many patients who are taking statins are treated at the same time with other medicines, it is important to know (although they are very rare) which medicines may increase the risk of adverse effects, particularly myopathy and rhabdomyolysis when used concomitantly with a statin (see Box 14.5). These medicines should be avoided when taking statins or, if absolutely necessary to receive them, caution is necessary.

Management of hypertriglyceridaemia

Hypertriglyceridaemia is an important risk factor/biomarker for cardiovascular risk. TG can be increased either because of inborn genetic errors of lipid metabolism or lifestyles or combination of both (see Box 14.6).

Box 14.6 Possible causes of non-genetically caused hypertriglyceridaemia

- Type 2 diabetes
- Obesity
- Excessive alcohol consumption
- Excessive soft drinks consumption
- Diet high in simple carbohydrates (sweets, honey, etc.)
- Some medications: peroral oestrogens, bile acid sequestrants, highly active antiretroviral drugs, some psychotropic drugs (phenothiazines, second-generation antipsychotics).

Box 14.7 Lifestyle interventions to lower TGs

- Reduce excessive body weight
- Reduce alcohol intake significantly
- Reduce carbohydrates intake significantly (particularly mono- and disaccharides)
- Take an omega-3 preparation (3–4 g/day)
- Increase everyday physical activity.

Box 14.8 Pharmacological treatment of elevated TGs

- Fibrates are the drugs of choice for treatment of hypertriglyceridaemia.
- If high TGs cannot be lowered to acceptable levels with a fibrate, a statin or an omega-3 preparation (3–4 g/day) can be added to decrease TGs further.
- In case of intolerance of fibrates, niacin or an omega-3 preparation (3–4 g/day) may be considered.

Elevated TGs can be reduced with lifestyles interventions much more successfully than elevated LDL-C (see Box 14.7). Therefore lowering of high TGs should always start with lifestyle interventions.

If with lifestyles intervention TGs cannot be lowered to acceptable levels (which is rarely the case) it should be continued but additional pharmacological treatment is necessary (Box 14.8).

How to influence low HDL-C

Low HDL-C is an independent and inverse CVD risk predictor. It can be increased predominantly with lifestyle interventions (Box 14.9).

If with lifestyles intervention HDL-C cannot be increased adequately, it should be continued but additional pharmacological treatment might be useful. However, the effects of available medicines to increase HDL-C are much more modest than the effects of medicines to lower LDL-C or TGs (see Box 14.10).

Lipids and some other parameters should be regularly followed in subjects with dyslipidaemia (Box 14.11).

Box 14.9 Lifestyle interventions to increase HDL-C

- Increase everyday physical activity
- Reduce dietary TFA intake
- Reduce excessive body weight
- Drink moderate quantities of alcohol (up to 20–30 g/day for men and 10–20 g/day for women)
- Reduce carbohydrates intake (particularly mono- and disaccharides).

Box 14.10 Pharmacological treatment for low HDL-C

- Niacin is at the moment the most efficient medicine to raise HDL-C.
- Statins and fibrates also raise HDL-C.

Testing lipids

How often should lipids be tested?

- Before starting lipid-lowering drug treatment, at least tow measurements should be made, with an interval of 1–12 weeks, with the exception of conditions where immediate drug treatment is suggested such as in acute coronary syndrome.

How often should patient's lipids be tested after starting lipid-lowering treatment?

- 8 (± 4) week after starting drug treatment.
- 8 (± 4) weeks after adjustments to treatment until within the target range.

How often should cholesterol or lipids be tested once a patient has reached target or optimal cholesterol?

- Annually (unless there is adherence problems or another specific reason for more frequent reviews)

Side effects of statins

Randomized control trials and meta-analyses suggest that statin side effects are rare, but post-marketing surveillance—and medical folk-lore—have raised some concerns.

Rhabdomyolysis occurs in perhaps 1 in 10,000 people, but aches and pains, usually with a normal muscle enzyme (creatinine kinase, CK) level, are common. Establishing a causal relationship is very difficult and the problem is compounded by media reports. If pain ceases when the statin is stopped and recurs when it is restated, options are to try a different statin or to start with a very small dose and increase it gradually.

Blood sugar may increase, especially in those prone to diabetes but in general the risk reduction associated with a reduction in LDL exceeds any harm from a modest rise in blood sugar.

Concerns about cancer and cognitive function have not been supported by objective evidence.

Monitoring liver and muscle enzymes

See Boxes 14.12 and 14.13.

How often should liver enzymes (alanine transaminase) be routinely measured in patients taking lipid lowering drug ?

- Before treatment.
- 8 weeks after starting drug treatment or after any dose increase.
- Annually thereafter if liver enzymes are <3 × ULN.

What if liver enzymes becomes raised in a person taking lipid-lowering drags?

If < 3 × ULN:

- Continuous therapy
- Recheck liver enzymes in 4–6 weeks.

If values rise to ≥ 3 × ULN:

- Stop statin or reduce dose, recheck liver enzymes within 4–6 weeks.
- Cautious reintroduction of therapy may be considered after alanine transaminase has returned to normal.

How often should CK be measured in patients taking lipid-lowering drugs?

Pre-treatment

- Before starting treatment.
- If baseline CK level > 5 × ULN, do not start drug therapy; recheck.

Monitoring

- Routine monitoring of CK is not necessary.
- Check CK if patient develops myalgia.

Increase alertness regarding myopathy and CK elevation in patients at risk such as: elderly patients, concomitant interfering therapy, multiple medications, liver or renal disease.

What if CK becomes raised in a person taking lipid-lowering drugs?

If > 5 × ULN:

- Stop treatment, check renal function and monitor CK every 2 weeks.
- Consider the possibility of transient CK elevation for other reasons such as muscle exertion.
- Consider secondary causes of myopathy if CK remains elevated.

If ≤ 5 × ULN:

• If no muscle symptoms, continue statin (patients should be alerted to report symptoms; consider further checks of CK).
• If muscle symptoms, monitor symptoms and CK regularly.

Legend:
ALT = alanine aminotransferace
CK = Creatine phosphokinase
ULN = upper limit of normal

Key reading

Reiner Z, Catapano AL, De Backer G, *et al*. ESC/EAS Guidelines for the management of dyslipidaemias: the Task Force for the management of dyslipidaemias of the European Society of Cardiology (ESC) and the European Atherosclerosis Society (EAS). *Eur Heart J* 2011; 32:1769–818.

Chapter 15

Managing blood glucose

Key messages

- Diabetes is a major CVD risk factor.
- Microvascular complications and other risk factors increase the risk associated with diabetes.
- Exercise and weight control can help to prevent the development of diabetes.
- It signals a need for intensive control of all risk factors.
- Targets for glycated haemoglobin (HbA1c) and other risk factors are defined in this chapter.
- Metformin is a first-line therapy.
- Statins are recommended in subjects over 40 years of age.

Summary

- Diabetes is a major risk factor for CVD, and CVD is a leading cause of death in people with diabetes, especially in the presence of microvascular complications and other risk factors. The ESC target HbA1c recommended for the prevention of CVD in diabetes is less than 7.0% (53 mmol/mol).
- Further reductions in HbA1c to a target of less than 6.5% (48 mmol/mol) may be useful in newly diagnosed patients.
- Hypoglycaemia and excessive weight gain should be avoided.
- A patient-centred approach to HbA1c targets (and choice of drugs) should be used, especially in patients with disease complications.

Cardiovascular prevention in people with diabetes

CVD is a leading cause of morbidity and mortality in people with diabetes. It can sometimes be prevented from developing by means of exercise and weight control.

The presence of microvascular complications and the presence of other risk factors increase the risk associated with diabetes. Intensive management of glycaemia in diabetes reduces the risk of microvascular complications (retinopathy, nephropathy, and neuropathy) and, to a lesser extent, CVD. The prevention of CVD in people with diabetes requires an intensified multifactorial intervention including the following:

- Assessment and management of all risk factors
- Blood glucose control as described in the remainder of this chapter
- BP control:
  - Multiple antihypertensive drugs are usually required to reach the target of less than 140/80 mmHg
  - ACEIs or ARBs should be included where possible
- Statins are recommended for diabetic people aged over 40 years, with higher doses of statins for diabetic patients with established CVD
- Antiplatelet therapy with aspirin is not recommended for people with diabetes who do not have clinical evidence of atherosclerotic disease
- Diabetic smokers should be given advice to quit and be offered assistance with smoking cessation.

Setting glycaemic targets

Glycated haemoglobin

HbA1c reflects the average plasma glucose over the previous 8–12 weeks. HbA1c was introduced into clinical practice in the 1980s and has become the cornerstone for the objective measurement of glycaemic control.

In 2011, the WHO recommended that measurement of HbA1c can also be used as a diagnostic test for diabetes, providing that stringent quality assurance tests are in place and assays are aligned to the international reference values. An HbA1c of 6.5% (48 mmol/mol) is recommended as the cut-off point for diagnosing diabetes.

HbA1c targets for people with diagnosed diabetes are based on the results of several large RCTs that are described in Box 15.1. Targets for HbA1c are included in local, national, and international guidelines for the management of diabetes. The 2012 joint ESC guidelines on cardiovascular disease prevention in clinical practice recommended a target HbA1c of less than 7.0% (53 mmol/mol), and this was repeated in the 2013 ESC guidelines on diabetes, prediabetes, and cardiovascular diseases developed in collaboration with the European Association for the Study of Diabetes (EASD). A lower target of less than 6.5% (48 mmol/mol) may be useful at diagnosis.

Implementation strategies for glycaemia management

Although guidelines establish general targets for HbA1c, it is important that these are discussed with the patient and an individual target is agreed. The target should take account of age, body weight, co-morbidities, and psychosocial factors, including employment (Table 15.1).

Targets should be less stringent in elderly patients, where the risks of hypoglycaemia are greater. Most patients with type 2 diabetes are overweight or obese, so drugs that do not cause weight gain may be preferred in many patients. Some patients will have co-morbidities where weight loss would be a benefit (e.g. sleep apnoea).

Box 15.1 Studies of intensive management of glycaemia in people with diabetes

Type 1 diabetes

Diabetes Control and Complications Trial (DCCT)

- In the intensive treatment group, HbA1c averaged 7.0% (53 mmol/mol) throughout the study
- Severe hypoglycaemia (requiring external assistance) and weight gain were common with intensive treatment
- Intensive control reduced retinopathy, nephropathy, and neuropathy during the study
- Intensive control reduced cardiovascular events on long-term follow-up.

Type 2 diabetes

United Kingdom Prospective Diabetes Study (UKPDS)

- In the intensive treatment group, HbA1c averaged 7.0% (53 mmol/mol) throughout the study
- Hypoglycaemia and weight gain were common with sulphonylureas and insulin
- Metformin reduced MIs in overweight patients during the study
- Intensive control reduced MIs and total mortality on long-term follow-up—a legacy effect.

Action in Diabetes and Vascular disease: Preterax and Diamicron Modified Release Controlled Evaluation (ADVANCE)

- In the intensive treatment group, the target HbA1c of less than 6.5% (48 mmol/mol) was reached after 3 years
- Hypoglycaemia and weight gain were uncommon with this slow titration of treatment
- Microalbuminuria was reduced during the study
- There was no apparent harm from intensive treatment
- Hypoglycaemia was a marker for patients with poor outcomes.

Action to Control Cardiovascular Risk in Diabetes (ACCORD)

- In the intensive treatment group, the target HbA1c of less than 6.0% (42 mmol/mol) failed to be reached
- Hypoglycaemia and weight gain were common with the rapid titration of treatment, including large doses of insulin
- Total mortality was increased and the study was halted prematurely
- Hypoglycaemia was a marker for increased mortality.

Table 15.1 Individual patient factors used to determine an appropriate glycaemic target

Approach to the management of hyperglycaemia	More stringent	Less stringent
Patient attitude and expected treatment efforts	Highly motivated, adherent, excellent self-care capacities	Less motivated, non-adherent, poor self-care capacities
Risks potentially associated with hypoglycaemia, other adverse events	Low	High
Disease duration	Newly diagnosed or short duration	Long-standing
Life expectancy	Long	Short
Important comorbidities	Absent	Severe
Established vascular complications	Absent	Severe
Resources, support system	Readily available	Limited

Most guidelines recommend an attempt at lifestyle interventions at diagnosis. In the UKPDS, intensive lifestyle change at diagnosis reduced HbA1c by up to 2%. This degree of improvement is difficult to implement in routine clinical practice, where more modest reductions in HbA1c will be obtained.

Antidiabetic drug therapy is usually started with a single drug, and guidelines generally agree that metformin is the preferred and most cost-effective first-line option. Occasionally, if the baseline HbA1c after lifestyle change is high (e.g. >9.0%) then patients will be started directly onto dual combination therapy.

If individual targets are not reached after 3–6 months of monotherapy then a second-line drug should be added as combination therapy. Again, if individual targets are not reached after another 3–6 months of dual therapy then third-line drugs should be added as triple combination therapy.

Following this, more complex combinations of oral antidiabetic drugs and injected treatments, including insulin, will be required. Insulin therapy should be considered as an early intervention for patients with significant hyperosmolar symptoms (thirst, polyuria, polydipsia) especially if they are losing weight.

Initial insulin therapy is usually started as basal insulin, and this can later be changed to more complex insulin strategies such as basal insulin plus a prandial insulin injection or twice-daily pre-mixed insulin injections.

A typical example of a guideline, which comes from Scotland, is shown in Fig. 15.1.

Therapeutic options

Lifestyle changes

Increasing physical activity and weight reduction through dieting improve glycaemic control and reduce other cardiovascular risk factors. At diagnosis, lifestyle changes may be sufficient to reach glycaemic targets without the need to introduce antidiabetic drugs.

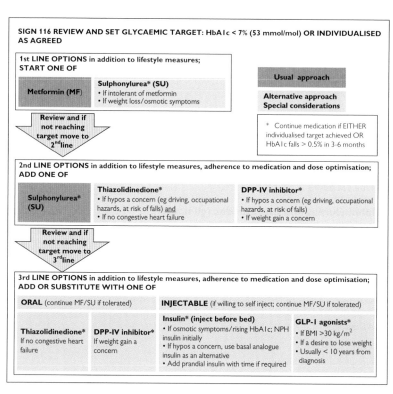

SIGN 116 REVIEW AND SET GLYCAEMIC TARGET: HbA1c < 7% (53 mmol/mol) OR INDIVIDUALISED AS AGREED

1st LINE OPTIONS in addition to lifestyle measures; START ONE OF

Metformin (MF)

Sulphonylurea* (SU)
• If intolerant of metformin
• If weight loss/osmotic symptoms

Usual approach

Alternative approach
Special considerations

Review and if not reaching target move to 2nd line

* Continue medication if EITHER individualised target achieved OR HbA1c falls > 0.5% in 3-6 months

2nd LINE OPTIONS in addition to lifestyle measures, adherence to medication and dose optimisation; ADD ONE OF

Sulphonylurea* (SU)

Thiazolidinedione*
• If hypos a concern (eg driving, occupational hazards, at risk of falls) and
• If no congestive heart failure

DPP-IV inhibitor*
• If hypos a concern (eg driving, occupational hazards, at risk of falls)
• If weight gain a concern

Review and if not reaching target move to 3rd line

3rd LINE OPTIONS in addition to lifestyle measures, adherence to medication and dose optimisation; ADD OR SUBSTITUTE WITH ONE OF

ORAL (continue MF/SU if tolerated)

INJECTABLE (if willing to self inject; continue MF/SU if tolerated)

Thiazolidinedione*
If no congestive heart failure

DPP-IV inhibitor*
If weight gain a concern

Insulin* (inject before bed)
• If osmotic symptoms/rising HbA1c; NPH insulin initially
• If hypos a concern, use basal analogue insulin as an alternative
• Add prandial insulin with time if required

GLP-1 agonists*
• If BMI >30 kg/m²
• If a desire to lose weight
• Usually < 10 years from diagnosis

Figure 15.1 Scottish Intercollegiate Guidelines Network (SIGN) Guideline 116: *Management of Diabetes.* Scottish Intercollegiate Guidelines Network (SIGN). *Management of Diabetes.* Edinburgh: SIGN; 2010. (SIGN publication no. 116).

In the recently completed Look Ahead study, a long-term randomized trial of lifestyle changes in people with type 2 diabetes, lifestyle changes reduced weight and improved fitness but had no effect on cardiovascular outcomes.

Metformin

Metformin is a biguanide that activates AMP-kinase and reduces hepatic glucose production. It is the usual first-line option.

Advantages

• Low cost
• Extensive experience
• No weight gain, possible weight loss
• No hypoglycaemia.

Disadvantages

- Gastrointestinal side effects:
  - Metallic taste in mouth
  - Diarrhoea
  - Abdominal discomfort
- Large tablet
- Lactic acidosis (rare).

Cardiovascular considerations

- Reduced MIs in UKPDS
- Withhold during acute heart failure.

Sulphonylureas and meglitinides (glinides)

Sulphonylureas and meglitinides close K_{ATP} channels on beta cell plasma membranes, releasing insulin.

Advantages

- Low cost (sulphonylureas)
- Extensive experience (sulphonylureas).

Disadvantages

- Weight gain
- Hypoglycaemia common.

Cardiovascular considerations

- In UKPDS, sulphonylureas as first-line therapy reduced MIs and total mortality on long-term follow-up
- In experimental models, some sulphonylureas inhibit ischaemic preconditioning.

Pioglitazone

Pioglitazone is a thiazolidinedione ('glitazone'), which activates the nuclear transcription factor PPAR-alpha. Rosiglitazone, another glitazone, was withdrawn because of a possible increase in MIs.

Advantages

- Increases insulin sensitivity
- Increases HDL-C
- Reduces TGs
- No hypoglycaemia.

Disadvantages

- Weight gain
- Fluid retention

- Increases fractures
- Possible increase in bladder cancer.

Cardiovascular considerations

- Reduced cardiovascular events in the PROactive study
- Contraindicated in heart failure because of renal fluid retention.

DPP-4 inhibitors

DPP-4 inhibitors ('gliptins') increase postprandial concentrations of incretin hormones, especially GLP-1. This increases insulin secretion and reduces glucagon secretion. Available drugs include sitagliptin, vildagliptin, saxagliptin, linagliptin, and alogliptin.

Advantages

- Weight neutral
- Hypoglycaemia uncommon
- Well tolerated.

Disadvantages

- Cost
- Long-term safety data awaited.

Cardiovascular considerations

- Sitagliptin, saxagliptin, and alogliptin had no effect on major adverse cardiovascular events (cardiovascular death, MI, stroke) in cardiovascular safety studies
- Saxagliptin increased hospitalization for heart failure.

SGLT2 inhibitors

SGLT2 inhibitors inhibit the reabsorption of glucose in the convoluted tubules of the kidney, promoting glycosuria.

Advantages

- Weight loss
- Can be used along with insulin therapy.

Disadvantages

- Cost
- Increase in genital fungal and bacterial infections
- Limited clinical experience to date
- Risk of volume depletion in vulnerable patients
- Longer-term safety data awaited.

Cardiovascular considerations

- Significant reduction in systolic blood pressure
- In the EMPA-REG OUTCOME trial empagliflozin significantly reduced major adverse cardiovascular events, total mortality, and hospitalization for heart failure.

Insulin

Insulin directly stimulates insulin receptors, increasing glucose disposal and reducing hepatic glucose output.

Advantages

- Extensive experience
- Generally inexpensive.

Disadvantages

- Weight gain
- Hypoglycaemia
- Subcutaneous injection or infusion.

Cardiovascular considerations

- In UKPDS, insulin as first-line therapy reduced MIs and total mortality on long-term follow-up.

GLP-1 receptor agonists

GLP-1 receptor agonists activate GLP-1 receptors, increasing insulin secretion, reducing glucagon secretion, slowing gastric emptying, and promoting satiety.

Advantages

- Weight loss
- Hypoglycaemia uncommon.

Disadvantages

- Cost
- Subcutaneous injection
- Gastrointestinal side effects:
  - Nausea
  - Vomiting
- Long-term safety data awaited.

Cardiovascular considerations

- Reduced cardiovascular events in observational cohorts
- Improve cardiac function in some animal models and preliminary human studies.

Other drugs

Acarbose inhibits intestinal alpha-glucosidase, slowing intestinal carbohydrate digestion and absorption. Reductions in HbA1c are modest, gastrointestinal side effects are frequent, and it is rarely used in European countries except Germany.

Orlistat is a gastric and pancreatic lipase inhibitor that reduces dietary fat absorption. When used in addition to antidiabetic drugs, including metformin, sulphonylureas, and insulin, it can reduce weight with slight improvements in HbA1c.

Hypoglycaemia

Hypoglycaemia is one of the main adverse effects of intensive glycaemia therapy in patients with type 1 or type 2 diabetes, especially when treated with insulin and/or sulphonylureas. Hypoglycaemia provokes an intense counter-regulatory hormonal response including:

- activation of the autonomic nervous system
- release of epinephrine (adrenaline)
- release of norepinephrine (noradrenaline)
- release of glucagon from pancreatic alpha cells.

The activation of the autonomic nervous system and the direct effect of neuroglycopenia on the central nervous system contribute to the symptoms and signs of hypoglycaemia that are described in Table 15.2. There can also be several serious cardiovascular consequences of hypoglycaemia, including MI and rarely sudden death.

Summary of managing blood glucose in type 2 diabetes

- The ESC target HbA1c recommended for the prevention of CVD in diabetes is less than 7.0% (<53 mmol/mol).

Table 15.2 Symptoms, signs, and cardiovascular effects of hypoglycaemia

Autonomic symptoms	Neuroglycopenic symptoms	Signs	Cardiovascular effects
Trembling	Difficulty concentrating	Sweating	Increased heart rate
Sweating	Confusion	Tremor	Widening of pulse pressure
Anxiety	Weakness	Bounding pulse	Increased cardiac output
Hunger	Drowsiness	Agitation	ECG changes, including QT prolongation
Palpitations	Visual change	Cognitive impairment	Arrhythmias, including atrial fibrillation
Nausea	Difficulty speaking	Drowsiness	Angina
Tingling	Headache	Coma	MI
	Dizziness		Cardiac arrest
	Tiredness		

- Further reductions in HbA1c to a target of less than 6.5% (<48 mmom/mol) may be useful at diagnosis.
- Hypoglycaemia and excessive weight gain should be avoided.
- A patient-centred approach to HbA1c targets (and choice of drugs) should be used, especially in patients with complex disease.

Key reading

Holman RR, Paul SK, Bethel MA, et al. 10-year follow-up of intensive glucose control in type 2 diabetes. N Engl J Med 2008; 359:1557–89.

Inzucchi SE, Bergenstal RM, Buse JB, et al. Management of hyperglycaemia in type 2 diabetes: a patient-centered approach. Position statement of the American Diabetes association (ADA) and the European Association for the Study of Diabetes (EASD). Diabetologia 2012; 55:1577–96.

Rydén L, Grant PJ, Anker SD, et al. ESC Guidelines on diabetes, pre-diabetes, and cardiovascular diseases developed in collaboration with the EASD: the Task Force on diabetes, pre-diabetes, and cardiovascular diseases of the European Society of Cardiology (ESC) and developed in collaboration with the European Association for the Study of Diabetes (EASD). Eur Heart J 2013; 34(39):3035–87.

The Action to Control Cardiovascular Risk in Diabetes Study Group (2008). Effects of intensive glucose lowering in type 2 diabetes. N Engl J Med 2008; 358:2545–59.

The ADVANCE Collaborative Group. Intensive blood glucose control and vascular outcomes in patients with type 2 diabetes. N Engl J Med 2008; 358:2560–72.

Zinman B, Wanner C, Lachin JM, et al. Empagliflozin, cardiovascular outcomes, and mortality in type 2 diabetes. NEJM 2015; 373:2117–28.

Chapter 16

Drug therapies to reduce risk: evidence and practicalities

Key messages

- Aspirin continues to be recommended for use in subjects with vascular disease but is no longer recommended in primary prevention, except perhaps in the highest-risk subjects.
- Perceived statin intolerance due to side effect effects (muscle, liver) is common but can usually be overcome.
- Muscle pain is common with statins but there is no easy way to establish causality. Rhabdomyolysis is rare.
- While no one drug is preferred in hypertension, ACEIs have a compelling indication in certain cases including established diabetes mellitus, established CVD and proteinuria.
- Mineralocorticoid receptor antagonists are used in heart failure and as reserve drugs in resistant hypertension.
- Beta blockers remain of value in secondary prevention and in the treatment of hypertension in certain cases.

Summary

- This chapter summarizes the indications for and side effects of the major classes of drugs used in CVD prevention, and offers guidance on specific statins.

Antiplatelet therapy

Aspirin

In primary prevention

- Aspirin is not recommended in primary prevention due to its increased risk of major bleeding.
- Aspirin is no longer recommended for people with diabetes who do not have clinical evidence of atherosclerotic disease.
- Aspirin can be considered in hypertensive patients without a history of CVD, with reduced renal function, or at high cardiovascular risk.

In secondary prevention

- In acute cerebral and coronary ischaemia, aspirin is recommended for prevention of recurrent cardiovascular events.
- In long-term secondary prevention after MI, stroke, or peripheral arterial disease, aspirin is of benefit and should be continued indefinitely.

Other antiplatelet therapies

Clopidogrel and prasugrel inhibit platelet aggregation through irreversible inhibition of the P2Y12 receptor. Prasugrel has faster onset with more potent platelet inhibition than clopidogrel (therefore carrying a slightly higher bleeding risk). Ticagrelor is a newer reversible inhibitor of the P2Y12 receptor and must be given twice a day.

Recommendations in acute coronary syndromes

In the acute phase and for the following 12 months, dual antiplatelet therapy with a P2Y12 inhibitor (ticagrelor or prasugrel) added to aspirin is recommended unless contraindicated due to such as excessive risk of bleeding.

Clopidogrel (600 mg loading dose, 75 mg daily dose) is recommended for patients who cannot receive ticagrelor or prasugrel.

Statins

Mechanism of action

Statins reduce serum LDL-C by reducing endogenous hepatic cholesterol production. This results in increased LDL receptor expression on hepatic cells increasing uptake of LDL by the liver and thus lowering serum LDL-C levels. Statins can also result in small increases in serum HDL-C levels (~5–10%) and reduce serum TG levels by ~20–45%. The common statins in clinical use and their pharmacokinetics are outlined in Table 16.1.

Why do the pharmacokinetics of statins matter in clinical practice?

- Certain statins should be taken at night (e.g. simvastatin, fluvastatin, and pravastatin) as these statins have a shorter half-life and endogenous production of cholesterol

Table 16.1 Pharmacokinetics of commonly used statins			
	Metabolism	Half-life (hours)	Hydrophilic
Simvastatin	CYP3A4	1–3	No
Atorvastatin	CYP3A4	13–30	No
Fluvastatin	CYP2C9	0.5–3	No
Pravastatin	Sulphation	2–3	Yes
Rosuvastatin	CYP2C9	19	Yes
CYP, cytochrome P450.			

is highest in the night-time period. Longer-acting statins such as atorvastatin and rosuvastatin therefore can be taken in the morning.

- The lipophilic statins (e.g. simvastatin) can cross the blood–brain barrier putatively causing insomnia and bad dreams. If this occurs, switch to a hydrophilic statin (e.g. pravastatin or rosuvastatin).

- All the statins with the exception of pravastatin are principally metabolized by the liver. Therefore pravastatin may be considered the most 'liver-friendly' statin.

- Caution is needed when CYP3A4 inhibitors (e.g. antifungals such as fluconazole, erythromycin/clarithromycin, and amlodipine) are concomitantly used with statins metabolized via the CYP3A4 pathway (e.g. simvastatin and atorvastatin). This can result in elevated statin levels and thus myopathy.

Dealing with common statin side effects

This area can cause a lot of confusion in clinical practice, often leading to inappropriate cessation of statin therapy and subsequent labelling of the patient as 'statin intolerant'. Being able to deal with statin side effects therefore is crucial.

Muscle side effects

Muscle side effects are one of the most commonly quoted side effects of statin therapy and are summarized in Table 16.2.

What to do if a patient develops muscle aches on statin therapy

- Take a clear history. It is important to distinguish symptoms from other causes of pain such as osteoarthritic joint disease or degenerative back problems. Ask about associated muscle weakness.
- Measure a CK level.
- If the CK level is normal, ask the patient to take a statin break for a week or so. Generally the symptoms will resolve quickly but will re-emerge if the patient recommences the statin. Options now include restarting statin at a lower dose or trying a low dose of another statin.

Table 16.2 Muscle side effects associated with statins			
	Definition	CK levels	Incidence
Myalgia	Muscle ache/discomfort but no weakness	Typically normal	No higher than placebo in RCTs. Up to 10% in clinical registries
Myopathy	Muscle discomfort also accompanied by weakness	Usually >10 times ULN	<0.01%
Rhabdomyolysis	Severe myopathy often with renal failure	Usually >40 times ULN	<1/3 the incidence of myopathy
CK, creatine kinase; ULN, upper limit of normal.			

- If it is a statin myopathy, the statin must be stopped and CK levels monitored until they return to normal. Statin myopathy tends to be more common with higher dose statins (in particular simvastatin 80 mg), in those with renal dysfunction, female, and the elderly.
- It does not mean statin therapy is now contraindicated and statin therapy may be retried at a lower dose at a later stage but ideally this should be done under specialist supervision.
- Rhabdomyolysis requires hospital admission with administration of intravenous fluid therapy. The risk/benefits of statin therapy in the future should be reviewed by a specialist.

Creatine kinase levels

It is worth measuring baseline CK levels. Some individuals may have a slightly elevated level at baseline particularly if they are very physically active or involved in contact sports. CK levels, however, do not need to measured routinely thereafter and only should be checked if the patient develops symptoms. Asymptomatic moderate rises in CK levels do not require any action.

Liver side effects

Less than 1% of patients will develop raised transaminases on statin therapy. This generally occurs in the first 6 months and is usually asymptomatic. Increases that are three times the upper limit of normal are considered significant but often resolve even if statin therapy is continued. However, if they persist after 1 month it is generally an indication for stopping the statin. Liver abnormalities are more common with the higher intensity statins particularly atorvastatin 80 mg.

Again, once transaminases return to normal the patient may be rechallenged with a lower-dose statin with monitoring of the liver function tests.

Non-alcoholic fatty liver is not a contraindication to statin therapy and may even be beneficial. Statins may also be used in most cases of chronic liver disease although liaison with a hepatologist may be advised alongside monitoring of liver function.

Modulators of the renin–angiotensin system

ACEIs/ARBs

Role in treatment of hypertension

Reviews of RCTs have shown that the main benefits of antihypertensive treatment are due to lowering of BP per se and are largely independent of the drugs employed.

However, there are some definite indications (and contraindications) for the use of ACEIs/ARBS in hypertension that are outlined in the Table 16.3.

- As a general rule of thumb, ACEIs should be used first line in preference to ARBs as they are supported by the largest body of evidence.
- ARBs are useful alternatives, however, when patients experience typical ACEI-related side effects (up to 10% of patients on ACEIs may experience a dry cough while <1% may develop angio-oedema).

Table 16.3 Indications and contraindications for the use of ACEIs/ARBs in hypertension

Indications	Contraindications
Diabetes mellitus	Pregnancy
Left ventricular hypertrophy	Bilateral renal artery stenosis
Proteinuria	Hyperkalaemia
Established CVD	Angioneurotic oedema[a]
Chronic renal disease	

[a] ACEIs only.

- The combination of ACEIs and ARBs in hypertension should be avoided due to the increased risk of side effects.

ACEIs/ARBs in secondary prevention

- ACEIs/ARBs are not just of value as antihypertensives but are also a keystone of secondary prevention measures even in those considered to be normotensive.
- Whilst they were originally found to have benefit in those with heart failure/ left ventricular dysfunction post MI they are now indicated in all patients post MI irrespective of left ventricular function.
- Evidence of benefit in stable CHD is not as clear cut but they may be considered in patients with features of increased cardiovascular risk (e.g. diabetes mellitus).
- ACEIs have also been shown to be of prognostic benefit in secondary prevention of stroke and also in those with peripheral arterial disease.

Dosing/uptitration

ACEIs/ARBs are often started at low doses (typically in hospital post MI) but it is important that they are subsequently uptitrated to 'evidence-based' doses, that is, those used in clinical trials (e.g. ramipril 10 mg once daily). Patients should be monitored for hypotension and renal function may also need to be monitored particularly in those with pre-existing renal dysfunction. However, an advantage of these particular drugs is that increasing the dose does not increase the risk of side effects such as cough.

Mineralocorticoid receptor antagonists

Spironolactone has been in clinical use for over 50 years and is a non-selective mineralocorticoid receptor antagonist. This can result in side effects including gynaecomastia, ED, and reduced libido in men and disturbance of the menstrual cycle in women. It can also cause hyperkalaemia in those with reduced renal function and should be avoided in those whose estimated glomerular filtration rate is less than 30 mL/min.

Eplerenone is a much newer selective mineralocorticoid receptor antagonist, thus avoiding the hormonal side effects associated with spironolactone and also due to its shorter half-life is less culpable in causing hyperkalaemia. However, the downside of its selective action is that it only has 60% of the potency of spironolactone.

Both drugs are useful in resistant hypertension (as a fourth-line agent) and are of prognostic benefit in chronic heart failure. Eplerenone has also been shown to be of benefit in patients post MI complicated by heart failure (in addition to standard therapy, namely ACEIs and beta blockers).

Beta blockers

Role in hypertension

- Beta blockers may still be used as first-line antihypertensives although this has been questioned in the past decade with some data suggesting a slight inferiority in preventing stroke.
- As beta blockers induce weight gain, have adverse effects on lipid metabolism, and increase the incidence of new-onset diabetes, they should be avoided in hypertensive patients with multiple metabolic risk factors (i.e. abdominal obesity, impaired fasting glucose, and impaired glucose tolerance) especially in combination with thiazide diuretics.

In secondary prevention

Beta blockers are of prognostic benefit post MI as a secondary prevention measure irrespective of the presence of hypertension or not and should be continued indefinitely. They are of particular benefit in patients who experience heart failure post MI and in those with asymptomatic left ventricular dysfunction.

Like ACEIs, they are often started at low doses post MI and it is important that is subsequently uptitrated as tolerated until the patient is 'beta blocked', that is, has achieved a resting heart rate under 60 bpm.

Side effects

There is often undue concern about beta blockers in patients with chronic obstructive airways disease (COPD). Whilst beta blockers are contraindicated in true asthma, most patients with COPD do not have bronchial hyper-reactivity and beta blockers can be safely used. If concerned, start with a trial of a low-dose, short-acting beta blocker (e.g. metoprolol 12.5 mg). Similarly, peripheral arterial disease is not a contraindication unless the patient has critical lower limb ischaemia.

Unlike ACEIs/ARBs, however, the risk of side effects does increase with increasing dose (including fatigue, cool peripheries, hypotension, and ED) which may have an adverse effect on patient adherence.

Key reading

Mancia G, Fagard R, Narkiewicz K, et al. (2013). 2013 ESH/ESC guidelines for the management of arterial hypertension: the Task Force for the Management of Arterial Hypertension of the European Society of Hypertension (ESH) and of the European Society of Cardiology (ESC). Eur Heart J 2013; 34:2159–219.

Perk J, De Backer G, Gohlke H, *et al.* European guidelines on cardiovascular disease prevention in clinical practice (version 2012). The Fifth Joint Task Force of the European Society of Cardiology and Other Societies on Cardiovascular Disease Prevention in Clinical Practice (constituted by representatives of nine societies and by invited experts). *Eur Heart J* 2012; 33:1635–701.

Reiner Z, Catapano AL, De Backer G, *et al.* ESC/EAS Guidelines for the management of dyslipidaemias: the Task Force for the management of dyslipidaemias of the European Society of Cardiology (ESC) and the European Atherosclerosis Society (EAS). *Eur Heart J* 2011; 32:1769–818.

Chapter 17

Identifying and managing psychosocial factors

Key messages

- Cardiovascular health depends on a balance of biological, psychological, and social factors.
- Psychosocial factors tend to cluster in people from low socioeconomic groups where the prevalence of CVD risk factors is high.
- Physicians and nurses are in an ideal position to screen for psychosocial risk factors and refer on to a psychologist or other psychology support.
- Assessment can be conducted using validated self-administered tools which generate a score and thus facilitate decision-making regarding referral.
- Measurement of psychosocial factors at different time points allows formalized evaluation of preventive initiatives from patients' and families' perspectives.

Summary

- This chapter identifies psychological and social factors that are associated with cardiovascular risk and describes how they can be practically assessed and managed.

Why do psychological and social factors matter?

Cardiovascular health depends on a balance of biological (e.g. BP and lipid profile), psychological (e.g. emotions and feelings), and social (e.g. having a supportive social network) factors. In reality this is a balance of 'risk' and 'protective' factors, rather than a complete absence of risk factors (see Fig. 17.1).

With respect to *psychosocial factors*, certain factors contribute to a higher risk of developing CVD and worsening of the clinical course and prognosis in patients with established CVD, and others have been demonstrated to be protective.

The following factors are associated with *increased cardiovascular risk*:

- *Acute stress*, that is, bursts of anger, severe anxiety, in patients with established CVD only

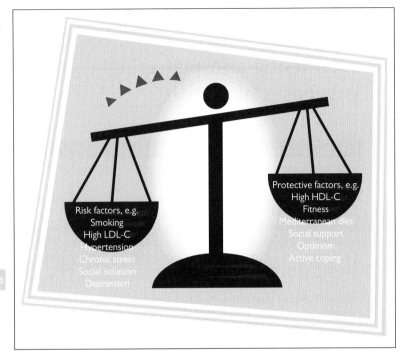

Figure 17.1 Cardiovascular health as a result of a balance between protective versus risk factors.

- *Low socioeconomic status*, that is, low educational level, low income, holding a low-status job, or living in a poor residential area
- *Social isolation and low social support*, that is, living alone, feeling isolated, or disconnected from others
- *Chronic work stress*, for example, lack of control over how to meet the demands of one's work, or receiving inappropriate rewards for one's effort ('gratification crisis'), and shift work, especially in men
- *Chronic stress in family life*, for example, conflicts, crises, and long-term stressful conditions, especially in women
- *Depression*, that is, feeling down, helpless, and hopeless; lack of pleasure in life, especially in combination with low social support
- *Anxiety*, especially generalized anxiety disorder and panic attacks
- *Hostility*, that is, extensive experience of mistrust, rage, and anger, and the tendency to engage in aggressive, maladaptive social relationships
- *Type D personality*, that is, an enduring tendency of a person to experience a broad spectrum of negative emotions (depressiveness, anxiety, irritability) and to inhibit self-expression in relation to others

- *Maladaptive coping with illness*, for example, extensive denial, but also catastrophizing, lack of motivation, and low self-efficacy
- *Severe psychiatric disorders*, such as schizophrenia and drug addiction.

Some of the aforementioned risk factors tend to cluster in the same individuals and groups (e.g. people of low socioeconomic status report chronic stress more often), together with more prevalent negative emotions (e.g. depression, anxiety, and hostility).

Increased CVD risk is mediated through the following behavioural and biological *mechanisms*:

- *Unhealthy lifestyle*, for example, more frequent smoking, unhealthy food choice, and less physical exercise
- *Low adherence* with lifestyle recommendations or cardiac medication
- *Financial barriers* to healthcare and healthy lifestyle
- *Inappropriate healthcare utilization*, for example, delay of help-seeking in case of emergencies
- *Psychobiological processes*, for example, alterations in autonomic function, the hypothalamic–pituitary axis, and other endocrine markers.

Together with unhealthy lifestyle and somatic risk factors, distinct psychobiological mechanisms affect haemostatic and inflammatory processes, endothelial function, and myocardial perfusion, thus resulting in subclinical manifestations of CVD and/or acute coronary syndromes (see Fig. 17.2).

Furthermore, certain medications for mental disorders (e.g. tricyclic antidepressants and neuroleptics) are associated with increased risk for cardiac arrhythmias and sudden cardiac death.

In contrast to the aforementioned risk factors, the following *protective psychosocial factors* for CVD have been identified:

- *Social support*, that is, a constant, caring relationship to one's spouse, friends, or family
- *Optimism, emotional competence*, and *high self-efficacy* as general coping resources
- *Adaptive coping with illness*, especially a tendency to get actively engaged in healthy lifestyles and adherence.

Protective factors are an important resource to cope with stress as well as somatic illness, once it is established. In particular, the capacity to change one's lifestyle is largely related to coping resources and social support (see also Chapter 8).

Assessment of psychosocial risk factors

Psychosocial risk factors can be assessed by:

- asking 'single-item' screening questions (see Table 17.1) during a consultation
- administering validated patient-reported outcome measure (PROM) questionnaires (see Table 17.2) during a consultation
- a standardized consultation.

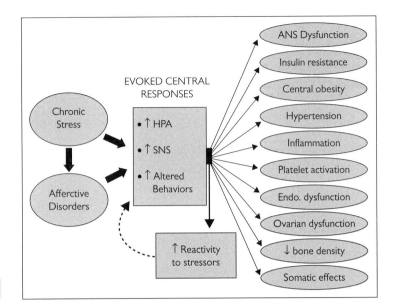

Figure 17.2 Psychobiological mechanisms by which chronic stress and affective disorders, such as depression, promote cardiovascular disorders.

Reprinted from *J Am Coll Cardiol*, 45/5, Rozanski A, Blumenthal JA, Davidson KW, Saab PG, Kubzansky L, The epidemiology, pathophysiology, and management of psychosocial risk factors in cardiac practice: the emerging field of behavioral cardiology, 637–51, Copyright (2005) with permission from Elsevier.

The first option is sufficiently reliable and the most time- and cost-saving way to assess psychosocial risk factors and is therefore highly recommended for clinical practice. In addition, this approach is helpful in building a *good rapport with patients*.

PROMs are frequently used in cardiac care as they produce standardized scores, which can be used to monitor quality and evaluate outcomes (see Chapter 22) and also for research. However, the use of PROMs should always be integrated into clinical decision-making and diagnostics, and should not serve as a replacement.

Standardized consultations, like the 'Structured Clinical Interview for DSM-5' (SCID-5), are restricted to the practice of psychiatrists and psychologists. The SCID-5 serves as a 'gold standard' for the diagnosis of mental co-morbidities, but it does not assess other risk factors like chronic stress, hostility, or type-D personality. It requires extensive training and is time-consuming; hence, it is of limited suitability for clinical practice.

How to conduct a consultation

- Allow enough time; a complete assessment of bodily and mental symptoms, and psychosocial factors, may take 20 minutes or longer.
- Be attentive and show empathy.

Table 17.1 'Single-item' screening questions recommended to be integrated into the consultation

Low socioeconomic status	Do you have no more than mandatory education? Are you a manual worker?
Work and family stress	Do you lack control over how to meet the demands at work? Is your reward inappropriate for your effort? Do you have serious problems with your spouse?
Social isolation	Are you living alone? Do you lack a close confidant?
Depression	Do you feel down, depressed, or hopeless? Have you lost interest and pleasure in life?
Anxiety	Do you frequently feel nervous, anxious, or on edge? Are you frequently unable to stop or control worrying?
Hostility	Do you frequently feel angry over little things? Do you often feel annoyed about other people's habits?
Type D personality	In general, do you often feel anxious, irritable, or depressed? Do you avoid sharing your thoughts and feelings with other people?

J. Perk, G. De Backer, H. Gohlke, *et al.*, European Guidelines on cardiovascular disease prevention in clinical practice (version 2012), *European Heart Journal*, (2012), 33,13, 1635–1701 by permission of Oxford University Press.

- Ask open-ended questions during the assessment and allow the patient time to answer.
- If psychosocial factors have not come up spontaneously in the consultation then work through the 'singe-item' questions or hand out questionnaires afterwards.
- Acknowledge the patient's personal view of their disease and psychosocial problems.
- Reflect back to your patient the key messages they express to demonstrate your understanding of their problem.
- Finish the consultation by giving a brief summary of what has been discussed. Ask your patient whether they would like to add anything, and confirm the key findings.
- Discuss the relevance of psychosocial risk factors with respect to health-related quality of life and prognosis, and close with shared decision-making regarding possible therapeutic consequences.
- A 'yes' for one or more items indicates a higher risk. Discuss with your patient the relevance of psychosocial factors with respect to their quality of life and medical outcomes.
- Physicians or trained nurses can conduct a consultation like this; however, if there is evidence of mental co-morbidities, either from the consultation or from the responses to the assessment questionnaires, a consultation with a *psychologist, psychiatrist*, or *psychotherapist* is strongly recommended.

Table 17.2 Patient-reported outcome measures (PROMs) suitable for routine screening of psychosocial risk factors

Risk factor	Questionnaire(name; number of items)	Time to administer (min)	Time for staff to score (min)	Clinical cut-off
Depression	Hospital Anxiety and Depression Scale (HADS); 7 items (depression)	5	1	Yes
	Prime MD Patient Health Questionnaire (PHQ); 9 items (depression)	5	1	Yes
	Beck Depression Inventory-II (BDI-II); 21 items	10	5	Yes
	Centre for Epidemiological Studies Depression Scale (CESD); 20 items (short form 15 items)	8	5	Yes
Anxiety	Hospital Anxiety and Depression Scale (HADS); 7 items (anxiety)	5	1	Yes
	Prime MD Patient Health Questionnaire (PHQ); 7 items (anxiety)	5	1	Yes
	State Trait Anxiety Inventory (STAI); 40 items (short form 16 items)	6–12	5	Yes
Anger/ hostility	State Trait Anger Inventory (STAXI); 44 items	10–15	5	Yes
Type D pattern	DS 14; 14 items	5	5	Yes
Social isolation	ENRICHD Social Support Instrument (ESSI); 7 items	5	1	Yes
Chronic work stress	Job Content Questionnaire (JCQ) ; 42 items	15	10	No
	Effort–Reward Imbalance (ERI), 23 items	10	10	No

Adapted from Albus et al., Screening for psychosocial risk factors in patients with coronary heart disease-recommendations for clinical practice. European Journal of Cardiovascular Prevention & Rehabilitation February 2004; 11:75–79.

Interventions

Interventions to manage psychosocial risk factors have beneficial effects on distress, quality of life, and functional status, even when added to standard prevention and reha- bilitation programmes. They can also impact on the course of clinical CHD, especially in patients who reach their behavioural goals.

The following interventions can be recommended in order to counteract psychoso- cial stress and support coping with illness:

- Supportive caregiver–patient interaction
- Enhancing social support
- Promoting physical exercise

- Counselling on psychosocial risk factors
- Stress management training
- Psychotherapy
- Medication
- Work reorganization.

Interventions should be individually tailored, based on the individual's risk consultation and treatment preferences. Gender-specific aspects (e.g. differences in family role, symptom presentation, coping, sexual problems, and health behaviour) should be considered, and interventions for men and women may be useful in many situations.

In patients at high CVD risk or with established disease, a multidisciplinary approach is highly recommended, which combines the efforts of physicians, nurses, dieticians, physical activity experts, social workers, and psychiatrists/psychotherapists. These interventions are available for in- and out-patients, and have been proven to moderate symptoms of anxiety and depression, as well as to impact favourably on health behaviour and cardiac prognosis (see also Chapter 8).

Frequent problems regarding the access and continuity of adequate care for psychiatric co-morbidities can be prevented by establishing 'integrated care', that is, the structured cooperation of physicians, nurses, and psychotherapists/psychiatrists. This kind of care is essential when patients are discharged from acute, hospital-based care to an ambulatory (e.g. out-patient, primary care, or community setting). Integrated care has been shown to significantly improve well-being and satisfaction with healthcare over and above standard settings.

Supportive caregiver–patient interaction

- A powerful tool to support behaviour change (see also Chapter 8)
- Enhances ability to cope with stress, illness, and moderate levels of depression and anxiety
- Helps to overcome resistance to treatment, often occurring in hostile patients, or in people with type D personality.

The following principles for a *supportive caregiver–patient interaction* can be recommended in order to address psychosocial risk factors:

- Spend enough time; even a few minutes more make a difference. In most situations, 10–20 minutes are satisfactory.
- Be friendly and attentive, control your own negative emotions.
- Use the 'ask—wait - answer' circle, and listen more than talk yourself.
- Acknowledge the patient´s personal view of their disease and social situation.
- Do not use protective buffering. Allow patients to explore and express their worries and anxieties.
- In patients with depressive symptoms, avoid being judgemental or pacifying. Express your willingness to build a supportive relationship.
- In patients with symptoms of anxiety, clarify concerns, and encourage step-by-step self-exposure to the anxiety-provoking situations (e.g. physical exercise).
- Explore further treatment options, such as a multidisciplinary programme, stress management training, psychotherapy, or medication, if appropriate.

- Agree a concrete plan.
- Ensure regular follow-up; initially once a week or every 2 weeks usually works well.
- Propose referral for psychotherapy and/or medication in the case of depressive and/or anxiety symptoms non-responsive to your efforts.

Enhancing social support

Adequate social support has been shown to be protective against virtually every kind of 'stressor' that may occur during a lifespan. Thus, interventions to enhance social support have a large potential to increase coping with illness and psychosocial stress.

The following interventions are recommended to increase social support in CVD patients:

- Involve spouses or other family members
- Self-help groups
- Heart sport groups
- Group psychotherapy.

Whichever method is selected, it should be agreed with the patient. In many cases, men like to involve their spouses, whilst women often prefer support from a close friend or other woman. The same is true for self-help groups, in which women tend to engage in a 'caring role' for their male group members, but do not feel supported in the same way as men.

Hostile patients, or patients with type D personality, often have reservations regarding self-help or heart sports groups. There is no point in trying to persuade or even urge such patients to join a group because this could seriously damage your rapport with the patient.

Promoting physical exercise

Regular physical exercise improves both bodily fitness and psychological well-being (see also Chapter 12). However, patients with psychosocial risk factors, especially depression and anxiety, are often reluctant to exercise due to low self-efficacy or because of irrational concerns. At the same time as attempting to build motivation to increase physical activity, remember to take potential barriers into account (see also Chapter 8). Patients often find heart sports groups to be very useful as a way of maintaining regular exercise, and at the same time, increasing social support.

Counselling on psychosocial risk factors

This kind of intervention can be performed on an individual or group basis. Counselling is *not psychotherapy*, and thus can be performed by trained nurses, psychologists, and social workers. Topics typically addressed in counselling interventions are psychosocial risk factors and coping with illness, but not mental co-morbidity. Basic principles of cognitive behavioural therapy (e.g. systematic problem analysis and cognitive reframing) are frequently used to help solve particular problems. At the same time, counselling groups can enhance social support.

In most cases, counselling is a part of a 'multidisciplinary intervention', thus, its duration is restricted to the underlying setting.

Stress management training

This intervention includes a collection of different therapeutic approaches, including *meditation, autogenic training, biofeedback, breathing techniques, yoga*, and *muscle relaxation*. The objective of stress management is to enhance coping resources by activating the body's own protective processes (e.g. vagus stimulation and lowering of muscle tension). In addition, self-assertiveness and distraction techniques are promoted.

Often, these techniques are combined so that patients can find out what works best for them. Integrating stress management techniques into everyday life requires training, support, and follow-up, otherwise maintenance in the long term is low (see also Chapter 8).

Psychotherapy

Coronary patients with *clinically significant depression, anxiety*, or *other adaptation disorder*, can be safely and effectively treated with psychotherapy. The following approaches are recommended:

- Cognitive behavioural therapy
- Interpersonal psychotherapy
- Psychodynamic therapy.

Psychotherapy in patients with somatic co-morbidities mainly aims at helping patients to cope with severe illness-related feelings and maladaptive cognitions, whilst at the same time offering a stable, supportive therapeutic relationship. In case of trauma-associated symptoms, further trauma-specific approaches should be added.

Psychotherapy can be performed on an individual basis, or in groups. Most patients prefer 'face-to-face' psychotherapy; however, depending on their treatment preference, many patients will also feel that group psychotherapy is an appropriate approach. In any case, it is most important to first assess the patient's preference regarding the setting of the intervention, and the gender of the psychotherapist, before they can be referred for psychotherapy.

In most situations, short-term psychotherapy (5–25 sessions, once a week) will be satisfactory to help patients adjust to their illness, and overcome episodic depressive or anxiety symptoms. In other, more complex situations like chronic depression or anxiety, hostility or the type D personality, longer, more intense interventions will be necessary.

Psychotherapy should be offered by trained professionals (psychologists or psychotherapists) only. Basic knowledge in cardiology is necessary for every psychotherapist, as it allows a mutual understanding of illness-related symptoms and somatic treatment options.

A crucial step is to motivate patients for psychotherapy. Many patients with established CVD fear the stigma of being labelled 'mentally ill'. Hence, it is most important to emphasize that symptoms of depression or anxiety are common in patients with CVD, and that modern cardiac care takes a holistic approach and aims at improving both bodily and mental well-being at the same time. Those not accepting psychotherapy should be followed closely and treatment offered again if symptoms persist for more than 4–6 weeks.

Medication

In case of clinically significant depression and/or anxiety, certain psychotropic medications are helpful in improving symptoms. The following medications are recommended in patients with CVD:

- *Serotonin reuptake inhibitors* (SSRIs; e.g. sertraline and citalopram), for treatment of depression, or generalized or phobic anxiety disorder
- *Mirtazapine* (second line, because of possible side effects), for treatment of depression
- *Benzodiazepines* (e.g. lorazepam), for treatment of acute anxiety—not longer than 2–3 weeks.

Tricyclic antidepressants (TCAs; e.g. amitriptyline), *tetracyclic antidepressants*, and *neuroleptics* (e.g. haloperidol) should be avoided, because of an increased risk of cardiac arrhythmias and sudden death. However, citalopram is also associated with increased QT prolongation in higher dosages. *St John's wort* should also be used with caution, because it can cause severe drug interactions with cardiac medications.

Patients should be informed of possible side effects, and precautions have to be taken not to dismiss possible problems with respect to *increased risk of bleeding* (SSRIs), *QT prolongation* (SSRI, TCA) or other *drug interactions* with cardiac medication (SSRI, TCA, St. John's wort).

Work reorganization

Shift work and chronic stress at work are common in patients with CVD. Changing from shift work to day work can be helpful, especially when patients report sleep disturbances.

In patients with chronic work stress, changing workplace in order to improve autonomy and increased control at work may result in less stress and a reduction in physiological stress responses.

However, these interventions cannot be easily prescribed, but should be discussed and implemented in cooperation with social workers and specialists in occupational medicine.

Key reading

Albus C. Psychological and social topics in coronary heart disease. *Ann Med* 2010; 42:487–94.

Albus C, Jordan J, Herrmann-Lingen C. Screening for psychosocial risk factors in patients with coronary heart disease – recommendations for clinical practice. *Eur J Cardiov Prev Rehabil* 2004; 11:75–9.

Bjanarson-Wehrens B, Grande G, Loewel H, *et al*. Gender-specific issues in cardiac rehabilitation: do women with ischemic heart disease need specifically tailored programmes? *Eur J Cardiovasc Prev Rehabil* 2007; 14:163–71.

Perk J, De Backer G, Gohlke H, *et al*. European guidelines on cardiovascular disease prevention in clinical practice (version 2012). The Fifth Joint Task Force of the European Society of Cardiology and Other Societies on Cardiovascular Disease Prevention in Clinical Practice (constituted by representatives of nine societies and by invited experts). *Eur Heart J* 2012; 33:1635–701.

Rozanski A, Blumenthal JA, Davidson KW, *et al*. The epidemiology, pathophysiology, and management of psychosocial risk factors in cardiac practice: the emerging field of behavioral cardiology. *J Am Coll Cardiol* 2005; 45:637–51.

Chapter 18

Putting educational strategies into practice

Key messages

- The concept of patient education has evolved from seeing the learner as an 'empty vessel' to fill with information to a more contemporary learner-centred approach that recognises prior learning and learner preferences.
- Educational resources should be tailored to health literacy levels.
- Practitioners should involve service users and carers in the development of educational resources for patients.
- Advances in technology offer exciting opportunities for the flexible delivery of learning materials.

Summary

- This chapter describes factors that influence learning, key educational theories, and gives examples of how theories can be applied in clinical practice.

Introduction

The education of patients, families, and colleagues is part of the day-to-day work of all health professionals. Yet little attention is given to the factors that influence the education process. Effective educational partnerships should be developed to support lifestyle change and medicines management. In this chapter, we describe factors that influence learning, outline relevant theories, and summarize tips about providing feedback.

Factors that influence learning

Knowledge alone is insufficient to change health behaviour. Nevertheless, education is central to the implementation of all interventions designed to promote health behaviour change and adherence to medicines. Focus is often given to educational content rather than the way that learning is delivered. Multiple factors influence the learning process (see Box 18.1). Communication-related behaviour change techniques (see Box 18.2) can be effective in supporting people with CVD to develop the knowledge, skills,

Box 18.1 Factors that influence learning

- *The physical environment*—temperature, noise level, light, and general comfort of the place in which learning is taking place.
- *The learner*—motivation and interest, health literacy level (see Fig. 18.1), feeling of safety and well-being, personal circumstances (physical and emotional status, e.g. level of worry, fatigue, and pain which impact upon concentration).
- *The topic to be learnt*—complexity and difficulty, relationship with existing knowledge, its relevance and usefulness in the short term and longer time-frame.
- *The time*—the time of the day, the time in the week, what has happened beforehand, and what will happen afterwards.
- *Previous experiences of learning*—has the person learnt in this way before, was it successful or not, confidence and self-belief, can they use what or how they learnt before to help them learn on this occasion?
- *The teacher or facilitator*—if the learning is being enabled by a 'teacher' how able are they to relate to the learner, their expertise, and teaching skills.
- *Significant others*—is the person learning with other people, who are they, and can they help or hinder the learning process?
- *Quality of learning resources*—is the learning supported by high-quality materials and learning resources, are they easily accessible and understandable to the learner?
- *Distractions*—for example, conflicting demands, competing pressures, procrastination, and the temptation to do other things.

and behaviours to make healthy lifestyle changes; all of the techniques have an educational component.

The influence of learner characteristics on educational initiatives

People from lower socioeconomic groups are more likely to have poor cardiovascular health and less likely to benefit from health promotion initiatives than those from more advantaged backgrounds. Health professionals who provide education to patients and their families can tailor provision to reflect the literacy and numeracy levels of their intended audience. In England, around one in six of the population has a literacy level equivalent to that of an 11-year-old. Health literacy, a term that describes attributes that go beyond literacy and numeracy alone, is defined as the capability, capacity, and opportunities that individuals have to identify, access, understand, appraise, and evaluate health information, and make informed decisions

Box 18.2 Communication-related behaviour change techniques

- Behavioural counselling
- Motivational interviewing
- Advice and information.

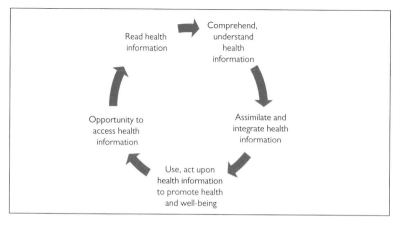

Figure 18.1 What is health literacy?

pertaining to it (see Fig. 18.1). It is particularly important and is a known determinant of health inequality. To encourage a meaningful level of patients and family engagement in decision-making about health it is important to tailor approaches and material at an appropriate health literacy level.

Health literacy is influenced by a number of factors, which operate at different levels (see Fig. 18.2). Effective communication skills and appropriately tailored health education resources can make health information more accessible to those who need it the most.

Implementing educational theory in clinical practice

In the past, the process of education has emphasized the role of the educator as an informer rather than a facilitator (see Fig. 18.3).

This view is now outdated in mainstream education and a more contemporary view places emphasis upon the learner and the process of learning. In the last decade, there has been an increased emphasis upon the concept of student-centred education, that fundamentally seeks to place the learner at the centre of the process (see Fig. 18.4). This approach aligns with current health policy, which aims to place patients and their families at the centre of healthcare provision.

The emphasis on person- and family-centred care (Box 18.3) and self-management (Fig. 18.5) further reinforces the idea of people, within their social networks, as active learners who seek information to inform the way they manage their own health and make decisions about treatments.

Self-management refers to a person's ability, within their life context, to live with and manage the day-to-day 'work' of living with a health condition. This may include the management of symptoms, medicines, lifestyle changes, and associated physical, functional, emotional, cognitive, and social limitations. As part of this process, a person

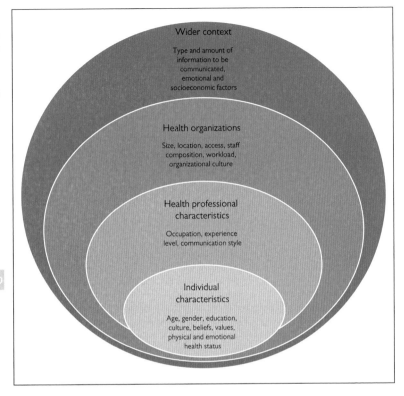

Figure 18.2 Factors influencing health literacy.

with CVD has to live with uncertainty about their health, respond to changes in their health status and manage their life in a way that provides an acceptable quality of life for them. The self-management process is dynamic, lifelong, and is learned through experience.

Learning theories

Learning theories present a set of linked ideas that describe how information is absorbed, interpreted, integrated, and retained during learning and provide a useful framework within which we can choose educational strategies to implement CVD prevention. Five overlapping theoretical ideas and related concepts are presented here that promote effective learning (see Fig. 18.6).

Active learning and student-centred learning

Active learning is a process in which the learner:

- actively engages with the topics and concept to be understood—may select information, solve a problem, plan a task

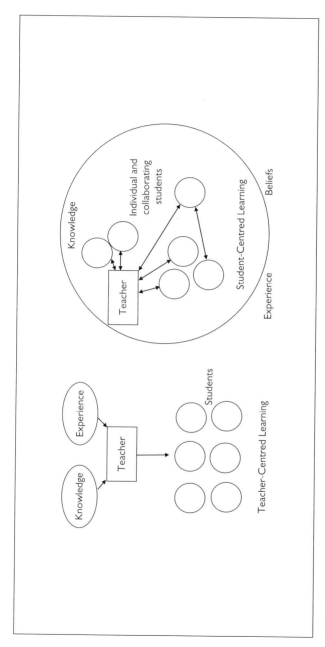

Figure 18.3 Educational approaches: informer vs facilitator.

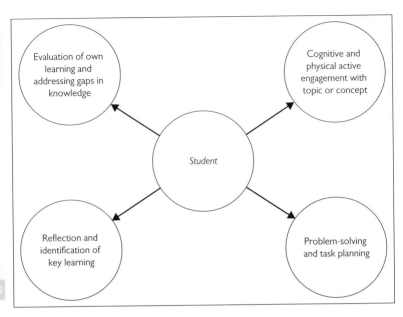

Figure 18.4 Student-centred learning.

- plans, acts, and reflects upon a learning task and identifies key learning from it
- self-assesses and actively evaluates their own abilities and level of understanding and takes responsibility for addressing gaps in their knowledge
- is cognitively, and perhaps even physically, engaged and active in the learning process.

Student-centred learning focuses on what the learner does rather than what the teacher does and:

- provides learners with control and choice in their learning; they have some influence on content, and the timing and delivery of learning
- may involve people learning independently, or with others; the educator often takes a guiding and facilitating role rather than an instructing one.

Box 18.3 Person- and family-centred care

Key concepts that underpin person- and family-centred care are:

- care, treatment, and support that is individualized and recognizes the life context of the recipient
- care, treatment, and support that is 'joined up' and coordinated across organizations
- care, treatment, and support that is compassionate but fosters independence through respectful collaboration.

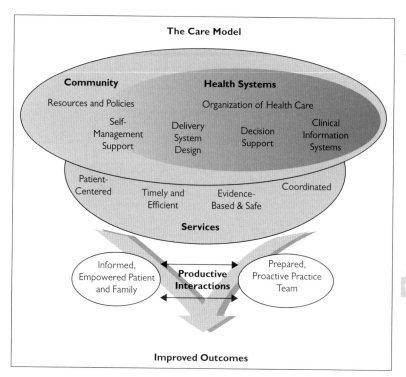

Figure 18.5 Self-management.

Wagner EH. Chronic disease management: what will it take to improve care for chronic illness? *Eff Clin Pract* 1998; 1:2–4.

Constructivism and experiential learning

Constructivism is probably the most influential educational approach currently in use:

- Learners use what they already know, together with the new ideas and concepts that they are taught, to construct their knowledge and understanding of the world.
- Learners must actively forge links and connections between new and existing knowledge to generate 'mental models' or schema to contextualize and understand them.
- Educators must assess what the learner already knows and understands at the outset, to avoid building on faulty foundations and embedding misconceptions.
- Learners are encouraged to construct their understanding through active experimentation, (planning, trying things out in practice, reviewing their experience, and relating it to their previous views and knowledge)—that is, active learning. This

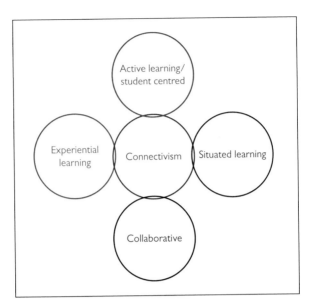

Figure 18.6 Theoretical ideas and concepts of learning.

idea of learning by experience also links to other theories developed across other disciplines, particularly psychology, which helps us to understand adherence to health behaviour change (see Box 18.4).

Experiential learning can occur in two ways:

- Through a direct encounter with the topic of learning, for example, on a course or in a training programme
- Through experiencing and reflecting on what happens to you in everyday life.

Box 18.4 Theory and health behaviour change

- Operant/social learning theory—behaviour is shaped through reward and punishment, role modelling, and observation of how others behave.
- Rational belief theory—rational beliefs are undesirable and irrational beliefs can be altered to optimize psychological health.
- Self-regulation theory—an individual is an active problem-solver and will behave in a way to formulate, trial, and appraise ways to attain a specific goal or state.
- Communications theory—communication is a complex process comprising several components and not simply the transmission of information.
- Health behaviour theories—explain differences across people, places, and situations with regard to different behaviours (e.g. transtheoretical model of change, health belief model, and theory of reasoned action; see also Chapter 8).

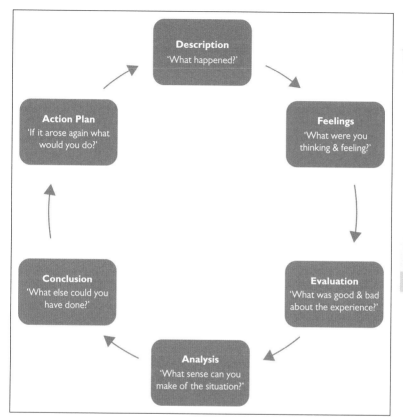

Figure 18.7 Reflective cycle.

Reproduced with permission from Gibbs, G. (1988) Learning by Doing: A Guide to Teaching and Learning, Oxford Centre for Staff and Learning Development, Oxford Brookes University, Oxford. This publication is available to download from https://www.brookes.ac.uk/OCSLD/Publications/

The idea of theory and practice informing one another in a continuous cycle (see Fig. 18.7) emphasizes the importance of reflection. Reflection is important for both learning and enhancing teaching and communication skills.

Situated learning

This viewpoint recognizes that learning is context dependent or 'situated':

- The learning environment needs to be relevant to the learning goals.
- The contextualization and application of knowledge to practice motivates learners who see its relevance.
- Situated learning theory also emphasizes social interactions with 'others' as learning does not take place in a vacuum.
- It challenges the view that learning can be readily transferred across new or different contexts.

In health professional education, emphasis is placed upon the need to provide real or simulated learning situations that expose the learner to the environments in which they will work.

Collaborative learning and the development of communities of practice

Collaborative learning

Collaborative learning is a powerful tool and we see that most people learn far more when they learn with others rather than in isolation.

Co-learners talk to each other, formulate questions, responses, and share experiences, using each other as sounding boards for new ideas. This may also involve giving and receiving feedback from peers.

Communities of practice

A group of people who share a commitment to a topic or set of interests and who are prepared to help and support each other with a view to learn from each other. This approach has been shown to be valuable in promoting learning between healthcare professionals and patients, who may be novices or experts at managing their health. It is thought to support evidence-based practice. Support groups for patients and families can also share some of these features. There is evidence that peer support telephone calls and lay-led self-management programmes can improve health and health behaviours.

Connectivism

The impact of accessible technology on how people learn is central to the theory of connectivism. It recognizes the importance of the social and cultural context of experiential learning but emphasizes the potential of the networks provided particularly by the Internet. Connectivism highlights:

- that learning involves connecting to information sources and hubs of specialized knowledge
- the need to nurture and facilitate connections and networks to support learning
- that the choice of what and when to learn is placed with, and controlled by, the learner.

All of the aforementioned educational theories can be used to inform CVD prevention and be applied to educational activities whether it be in a formal (e.g. in a classroom with students, workshop with patients, or families in a cardiac rehabilitation setting) or in a less formal setting (e.g. a consultation with a patient and spouse, an out-patient appointment, or a chat by the hospital bed). Box 18.5 lists some key points to consider applying when you are teaching colleagues, patients, and their families.

Providing feedback

It is important to develop an action plan which incorporates goal setting to support patients and families with lifestyle change and medication management in CVD prevention initiatives. The ongoing evaluation of such plans requires personalized feedback about progress (see Box 18.6).

Busy health professionals all face constraints on the time available to educate patients and their families. This makes the planning process very important, particularly as

Box 18.5 Key points arising from learning theories to consider when conducting educational activities

- Don't just inform! Actively engage the learner, and significant other, in their learning.
- Provide opportunities for the learner to put learning into practice (e.g. active learning tasks).
- Give a choice about when, how, and at what pace learning happens.
- Support the learner to take responsibility for managing their own learning and evaluating their own knowledge.
- Recognize the influence of culture, literacy level, and language on setting the learning expectations and experiences of learners.
- Clarify what is already known or understood by the learner (and identify misunderstandings/misperceptions).
- Aid patients to develop mental models that allow them to connect what they know with what they experience, and with what they are learning anew.
- Enable learners to de-brief and reflect upon their own experiences and learning.
- Consider how learners, whether professionals or patients, are supported to transfer and apply knowledge gained in clinics, hospital, or college to their home or working environments.
- Recognize the importance of the 'significant others' who are part of the learner's environment.
- Enable the learner to learn with others, either face-to-face, or online.
- Support learners (and healthcare professionals) to share their experiences and knowledge. Patients who have become 'expert' in living with their health condition may support those who are 'novices'.
- Recognize that information and communication technology provides an innovative delivery mechanism for health information and education; however, patients may need support to be able to find helpful and accurate material and make useful connections online.
- Recognize that connectivity supports the development of online materials that can be navigated and explored in ways chosen by the learner.

patients and families often report unmet health information needs. When preparing for a consultation, prioritize the information that you need to convey (see Fig. 18.8) and think about different ways of delivering it.

Building educational content

Educational content can be visualized as a 'spiral curriculum' (see Fig. 18.9) which is designed so that the study of a topic is repeated several times during a course of teaching and each time at greater depth, difficulty, and complexity. This approach of repeating cycles has also been used to improve induction programmes, where it is common

Box 18.6 Top tips for effective feedback

One example might be giving feedback about progress made with goals set within an individualized action plan as part of cardiac rehabilitation. Feedback will be most productive when it is:

- *timely*—connected with the experience of learning
- *specific*—uses the learner's own experience to situate the feedback
- *honest*—really communicates the reality of the situation
- *constructive*—doesn't just indicate what is wrong but suggests how to improve it in the future
- *prompts a dialogue*—is not a one-way communication but initiates personal reflection and a conversation and exchange
- *verbal and written*—if written feedback is provided, its impact can be increased if the learner has the opportunity to talk about it, and if verbal feedback is provided, encouraging the learner to write something down is beneficial
- *balanced praise and criticism*—positive feedback to reinforce existing good practice together with more critical feedback indicating where changes can be made in the future
- *encouraging*—delivered in a way that motivates and encourages the learner to want to act on the feedback and builds their confidence and self-belief.

to overload people with too much detail and too much information before they are really ready for it. The same may be true when giving patients information about their illness or treatment.

Using appropriate media to convey knowledge

The most effective way to improve CVD knowledge and behavioural outcomes is through the use of a combination of learning and teaching approaches to suit a variety of learning styles, including:

- written
- audiovisual
- pictorial material.

'Need to know and do'
Important information about diagnosis, key treatment, and management of prescribed medications

'Nice to know and do'
Information that may be covered but can wait for a second consultation

'Not necessarily now, do later'
Information about additional services that could be provided using leaflets, booklets, or web-based resources

Figure 18.8 Prioritizing information to communicate.

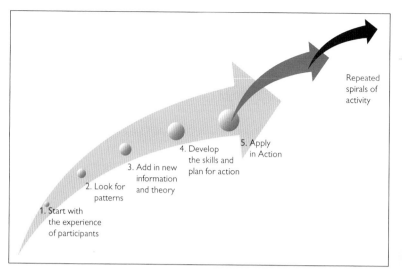

Figure 18.9 Activity taking place in repeated learning spirals.

A combination of written and verbal information is more effective than verbal information alone. The use of tape recordings or written summaries has been reported as a useful adjunct to support information provision and education in medical consultations.

In summary, health professionals play a key role as educators for patients and their families. The process of learning is influenced by the characteristics of the teacher, learner and the environment. The multiple ways of communication afforded by today's information technology presents us with many exciting opportunities for innovative patient education. The effective self-management of lifestyle and cardioprotective medicines, by patients and their families, is fundamental to prevention. Through the careful development of appropriate health information resources, delivered using sound educational strategies, we have the potential to further maximize upon our efforts to reduce the burden of CVD.

Key reading

Driscoll MC. *Psychology of Learning for Instruction* (2nd ed). Needham Heights, MA: Allyn & Bacon, 2000.

Kolb DA. *Experiential Learning: Experience as the Source of Learning and Development.* Englewood Cliffs, NJ: Prentice-Hall, 1984.

Kop R, Hill A. Connectivism: learning theory of the future or vestige of the past. *Int Rev Res Open Distance Learn* 2008; 9(3):1–13. http://www.irrodl.org/index.php/irrodl/article/view/523/1103

Lave J, Wenger E. Learning and pedagogy in communities of practice. In Leach, J, Moon B (eds) *Learners and Pedagogy.* London: Paul Chapman Publishing, 1999:21–33.

Sorensen K, Van Den Brooke S, Fullam J, et al. Health literacy and public health, a systematic review and integration of definitions and models. *BMC Public Health* 2012; 12:80.

Part 3

Setting up preventive cardiology initiatives

Chapter 19

The global care pathway and how it works in practice

The care pathway shown in Fig. 19.1 identifies the stages to follow when an individual presents for a cardiovascular risk assessment, whatever the category of risk they fall under. These stages apply irrespective of the setting in which cardiovascular prevention will be implemented. Whereas patients with an acute event are most likely to be identified in hospital, those at high cardiovascular risk with multiple risk factors or with diabetes are more likely to be identified by their general practitioner (GP).

Wherever patients present, they should be assessed and their risk categorized. Preventive initiatives, wherever they are set up, should work towards targets and within an interdisciplinary framework providing care at the convenience of patients and their families.

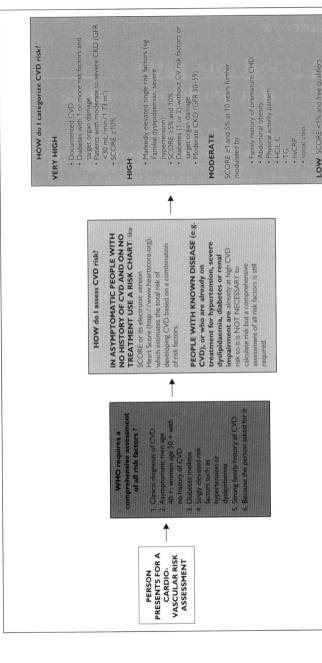

PERSON PRESENTS FOR A CARDIOVASCULAR RISK ASSESSMENT

WHO requires a comprehensive assessment of all risk factors?

1. Clinical diagnosis of CVD
2. Asymptomatic men age 40+ women age 50+ with no history of CVD
3. Diabetes mellitus
4. Singly elevated risk factors such as hypertension or dyslipidaemia
5. Strong family history of CVD
6. Because the person asked for it

HOW do I assess CVD risk?

IN ASYMPTOMATIC PEOPLE WITH NO HISTORY OF CVD AND ON NO TREATMENT USE A RISK CHART: like SCORE or its electronic version Heart Score (http://www.heartscore.org), which estimates the total risk of developing CVD based on a combination of risk factors.

PEOPLE WITH KNOWN DISEASE (e.g. CVD), or who are already on treatment for hypertension, severe dyslipidaemia, diabetes or renal impairment are already at high CVD risk so it is NOT NECESSARY to calculate risk but a comprehensive assessment of all risk factors is still required.

HOW do I categorize CVD risk?

VERY HIGH:
- Documented CVD
- Diabetes with 1 or more risk factors and target organ damage
- Patients with moderate to severe CKD (GFR <30 mL/min/1.73 m^2)
- SCORE ≥10%

HIGH:
- Markedly elevated single risk factors (eg. Familial dyslipidaemias, severe hypertension)
- SCORE ≥5% and 10%
- Diabetes (1 or 2) without CV risk factors or target organ damage
- Moderate CKD (GFR 30–59)

MODERATE:
SCORE ≥1 and 5% at 10 years further modulated by
- Family history of premature CHD
- Abdominal obesity
- Physical activity pattern
- HDL-C
- TG
- hsCRP
- social class

LOW: SCORE <1% and free qualifiers

Figure 19.1 Global care pathway.

WHAT are the targets?

- No exposure to tobacco in any form
- Healthy diet low in saturated fat with a focus on wholegrain products, vegetables, fruit and fish
- 2.5 to 5 hours of moderately vigorous physical activity per week or 30–60 minutes most days
- BMI 20–25. Waist circumference <94 cm (men) or <80 cm (women)
- BP <140/90
- Lipids:
  - Very high risk LDL-C<1.8 mmol/L or >50% reduction
  - High risk LDL-C<2.5 mmol/L
  - Low to moderate risk LDL-C <3 mmol/L
  - HDL-C no target but >1 mmol/L in men and >1.2 mmol/L in women indicates lower risk
  - Triglycerides no target but <1.7 mmol/L indicates lower risk and higher levels indicate a need to look for other risk factors
- Diabetes: HbA1c <7% and BP <140/80

WHERE should CVD prevention be offered?

- Healthy lifestyles should be promoted from childhood
- Life-long prevention through avoidance of all forms of tobacco, healthy eating and physical activity should be initiated and coordinated by the primary care team
- Hospital- or community-based multidisciplinary teams should be developed and promoted to deliver primary prevention for people at high CVD risk
- Hospital patients with CVD should be discharged with a clear guideline-based risk factor management plan and offered participation in a cardiovascular prevention and rehabilitation programme
- Families of vascular and high risk patients should all be included in preventive care
- The risk status of relatives of persons with premature CVD should be systematically assessed and managed

Figure 19.1 Continued

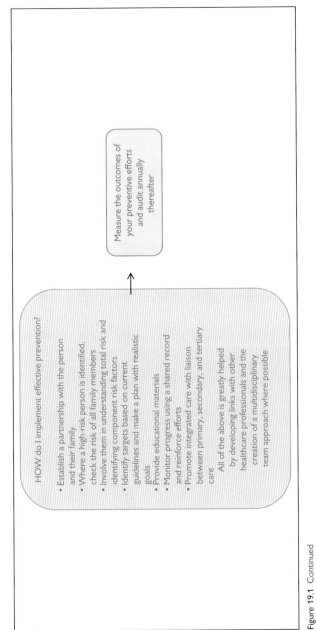

HOW do I implement effective prevention?

- Establish a partnership with the person and their family
- Where a high-risk person is identified, check the risk of all family members
- Involve them in understanding total risk and identifying component risk factors
- Identify targets based on current guidelines and make a plan with realistic goals
- Provide educational materials
- Monitor progress using a shared record and reinforce efforts
- Promote integrated care with liaison between primary, secondary, and tertiary care

  All of the above is greatly helped by developing links with other healthcare professionals and the creation of a multidisciplinary team approach where possible

Measure the outcomes of your preventive efforts and audit annually thereafter

Figure 19.1 Continued

Chapter 20

Examples of initiatives in different care settings: starting preventive and rehabilitative care in hospital

Key messages

- Prevention and rehabilitation should start in the acute setting prior to hospital discharge.
- A clinical evaluation and risk assessment are indispensable following a cardiac event and will determine how to tailor a programme of prevention and rehabilitation.
- Information-giving in hospital should be simple and clear given the potentially limited ability to absorb information immediately after a vascular event.
- The hospital healthcare team, led by the cardiologist, should include professionals with the necessary multidisciplinary expertise and this team should consistently reinforce the need for attendance at a structured out-patient programme of prevention and rehabilitation.
- Effective discharge planning should be facilitated with the use of a clear communication in the form of a comprehensive letter directed at the GP, patient, the family, and the care-givers.
- Structured prevention and rehabilitation programmes should start early after hospital discharge, include core components, and conform to minimal standards.

Summary

- This chapter describes the principles of initiating preventive and rehabilitative care during hospitalization following a vascular event.

Introduction

After experiencing an acute event and revascularization procedure, patients should begin a structured programme of prevention and rehabilitation as soon as possible after admission to hospital. This programme should continue in an out-patient, in a residential- or home-based setting. It will be attended remotely, depending on clinical, administrative, and logistic reasons and personal patient preferences after discharge from hospital.

In the acute stage, the programme should comprise the following:

- Post-acute clinical evaluation and risk assessment
- General counselling: basic information and reassurance
- Psychological and social support
- Early mobilization and physical activity counselling
- Discharge planning, including referral to out-patient care and a structured programme of cardiovascular prevention and rehabilitation.

The acute phase in hospital is therefore the first step in a programme of preventive cardiology. A system should be in place that ensures that every eligible cardiovascular patient has access to an individualized programme and, where possible, group education and discussion while they are an in-patient.

In accordance with recent European statements, a secondary prevention programme should include the following core components:

- Clinical and risk assessment
- Physical activity counselling
- Prescription of exercise training
- Smoking cessation
- Diet/nutritional counselling
- Weight control management
- BP management
- Lipid management
- Psychosocial management
- Vocational support.

Whilst secondary prevention programmes should integrate all of the core components because they are applicable to all cardiovascular conditions, these components should be tailored to individual needs, according to specific clinical conditions.

The expected outcomes of these interventions are improved clinical stability and symptom control, reduced overall cardiovascular risk, higher adherence to pharmacological advice, and better health behaviour profile, all leading to superior quality of life, social integration, and improved prognosis.

Post-acute clinical evaluation and risk assessment

This should include a review of clinical history, including the physical activity level before the acute event, evaluation of actual clinical signs and symptoms, physical and functional examination, as well as diagnostics such as ECG and ECG monitoring, echocardiography, laboratory examinations, and coronary angiogram, and can be regarded as clinical routine.

The initial medical assessment should identify major cardiovascular risk factors and severity of the disease. This assessment is indispensable as it will decide both the short- and long-term prognosis, the core components of the individual preventive strategy at the start of the structured programme of prevention and rehabilitation.

To be screened for and appropriately treated

- Severity of CAD
- Myocardial damage
- Existence of arrhythmias
- Coexisting co-morbidities.

The whole therapeutic team should be well informed of the clinical status and of all remaining risk factors. This is a prerequisite for appropriate counselling and for getting the patient safely mobilized.

General counselling: basic information and reassurance

During their hospital stay, patients want and need information on a range of topics, including advice about their illness, its causes, course, and prognosis, treatment, necessary lifestyle change, activity levels, and how to manage their condition. Interventions correcting cardiac misconceptions improve knowledge and reduce stress for the patient, their partner, and their family. Individual patient's needs for information will need to be tailored, depending on gender, ethnicity, education, age, and social status.

In the acute stage in hospital, patients' receptivity and ability to understand and absorb detailed and complex information may be limited by physical illness and psychological and cognitive (memory and attention) reactions. Information given should be clear, simple, and based on the individual and family needs. Reassurance, support, and empathy should underpin all discussions.

The healthcare team should base counselling content on the detailed knowledge of the patient's risks and risk factors as well as on the social environment. The team should hold regular meetings to discuss individual patients and their problems, and to ensure an integrated therapeutic multidisciplinary team approach. The team should include members with the necessary expertise (e.g. dietetics, diabetes, and cardiology).

As medical and social issues are always interrelated and influence one another, it is essential to consider potential facilitators and barriers in an individual's social life when giving advice on medication and lifestyle changes.

Box 20.1 shows the topics to cover in counselling during this acute phase. Remember to adapt counselling to patients' pre-existing knowledge and individual needs.

It is very important during this in-hospital phase that the whole healthcare team (led by the cardiologist) reinforces the importance of participating in the structured prevention and rehabilitation programme after hospital discharge to both the patient and to key family members (e.g. spouse and offspring). In addition to initiating good lifestyle and risk factor treatment, the counselling should also include as an imperative initiating the occupational and social reintegration of the patient.

- Offer reassurance and explanation of cardiac condition, treatment, and procedures.
- Give general and individualized information on CAD, acute MI, and their consequences.
- Provide information on how to recognize and interpret signs and symptoms of ischaemia, heart failure, and arrhythmias.
- Agree an action plan with the patient and family to ensure early response to warning symptoms.
- Advise on acute and chronic treatment, and type and doses of medications, highlighting the importance of adherence.
- Reinforce cardiovascular prevention—the identification and modification of risk factors should be addressed in general and focused on the individual's needs.
- Explain the in-patient activity programme, advantages, related risks, warning symptoms, and monitoring modus operandi.
- Give information on how to progressively resume physical, sexual, and daily living activities (including driving and return to work).
- Explore the potential impact on social life, the family, and personal relationships, and assess social support/isolation.
- Social support.

Psychological and social support

Psychological care and counselling should start as early as possible, and then continue during the structured prevention and rehabilitation programme as appropriate. Early identification of psychosocial problems and intervention in those most at risk can reduce psychological distress, hospital readmission rates, and anxiety and depression scores. Psychosocial interventions may also reduce symptoms like angina, and support clinical recovery as well as return to work.

**Pre-hospital discharge interventions that may help patients'
and family members' knowledge and involvement**

- Brief advice for smoking cessation
- Audiotapes
- Video tapes
- Post-discharge telephone counselling plan.

Mobilization and physical activity counselling

During the in-hospital phase, the patient takes the first step to regaining physical independence and self-confidence. The primary purpose of early mobilization is to safely prevent the risks and complications of prolonged immobilization, which include almost

- Positioning prone or side-to-side in bed
- Use of continuous lateral rotating therapy beds
- Breathing exercises
- Passive and active range of motion
- Dangling
- Moving out of bed to a chair
- Movement in the bed to an upright position
- Ambulation
- Ambulation using staircases
- Tilting on a table
- Use of active resistive exercise
- Use of electrical muscle stimulation.

all organ systems and may lead to severe psychological consequences. Additional goals are to accelerate remobilization, to regain cardiovascular fitness and functional abilities, and to increase comfort and psychological well-being. Early remobilization therefore is considered as common practice in the care of hospitalized patients and may be implemented through a broad range of activities. Box 20.2 describes examples of activities for early mobilization, while Box 20.3 provides recommendations on how to manage early remobilization in clinical practice.

Effective discharge planning should ensure a seamless move from hospital into the home environment and care services provided beyond acute care. To do this it needs to coordinate and integrate the expertise of several different disciplines working across primary and secondary medical care and in the social services.

Hospital discharge requires good communication between healthcare providers (physician or dedicated nurse) and patients and families. A detailed discharge letter

Box 20.3 Recommendations on how to manage early remobilization in clinical practice

- Prescribe early mobilization taking into account type and dosage (intensity, duration, frequency) of the intervention.
- Regularly monitor heart rate, breathing activity, and BP, as well as signs and symptoms of ischaemia, heart failure, and arrhythmias.
- Adjust the physical activity intervention with respect to type and dosage according to the individual patient condition and response to exercise.
- Adopt a stepwise increase in dosage in an individualized fashion and include additional types of interventions and exercise programmes (see Box 20.2).
- Use a multidisciplinary approach with a frequent interaction between healthcare providers (physician, nurse, physiotherapist, and so on).
- Discharge planning.

Box 20.4 Example of a discharge letter

DATE OF ADMISSION:
DATE OF DISCHARGE:

DIAGNOSIS:
1. Admitting diagnosis:_____
2. Secondary diagnosis:_____

PATIENT MEDICAL HISTORY:
☐ Family history:_____
☐ Social history: _____
☐ Allergies: _____
☐ Brief medical history: _____
☐ History of present illness: _____

HOSPITAL STAY:
☐ Physical examination at admission: _____
☐ Diagnostic procedures performed: _____
☐ Results obtained:_____
☐ Hospital course and treatment:_____
☐ Counselling/advice_____

DISCHARGE:
☐ Discharge diagnosis:_____
☐ Condition on discharge and active problems (if appropriate):_____
☐ Functional status at discharge:_____
☐ Discharge medications:_____
☐ Discharge instructions: _____
☐ Cardiovascular risk profile: refer to HeartScore, source
   http://www.heartscore.org
☐ Discharge diet (if appropriate):_____
☐ Discharge physical activity recommendation: _____

☐ Preventive goals:
• Stop smoking
• LDL cholesterol <70 mg/dL (or 50% reduction when not possible)
• Weight loss goal (if appropriate): ____kg
• Waist circumference <102 cm (male) <88 cm (female)
• Non-diabetics:
   • Blood pressure 140/90 mmHg
• Diabetics:
   • Blood pressure <140/85 mmHg
   • Glycated haemoglobin <7%

REFERRAL AND FOLLOW-UP
☐ In/out-patient, cardiovascular prevention and rehabilitation programme:

Why: _____
When: _____
Where: _____

supports the transition from hospital to home. Standardized templates for discharge letters and other communications are available to promote efficiency and consistency of practice. An example of a discharge letter template is provided in Box 20.4.

Referral to structured cardiovascular prevention and rehabilitation programme

Early referral to a structured cardiovascular prevention and rehabilitation programme is an imperative for all patients: automatic referral using electronic patient records or standard discharge orders in combination with individual and personal information and reinforcement appears to be the best way to get a high attendance at these programmes. In reality, the choice of programme setting in most countries is driven by availability, but also depends on local health service provision, the type and support of health insurance and pension schemes, and the government. Whereas most patients are suitable for out-patient programmes, the following criteria may be regarded as a basis for choosing a residential/hospital-based programme over an out-patient programme:

- Persistent clinical instability, or serious and clinically unstable concomitant diseases
- Clinically unstable patients with advanced heart failure (New York Heart Association class III–IV, needing intermittent or continuous drug infusion and/or mechanical support)
- A recent heart transplantation and ventricular assist device implantation
- Discharged very early after the acute event and with remaining high risk of clinically instability and/or unstable comorbidities
- Unable to attend a formal out-patient programme for any logistic reasons.

Independent of the setting for such programmes, their effect and success is strongly dependent on content, intensity, and patient adherence. Programmes should follow minimal standards and include core components as mentioned earlier in this chapter. Some countries have developed their own standards and core components. See, for example, the United Kingdom example (http://www.bacpr.com/resources/15E_BACPR_Standards_FINAL.pdf).

Key reading

Amidei C. Mobilization in critical care: a concept analysis. *Intensive Crit Care Nurs* 2012; 28:73–81.

Bjarnason-Wehrens B, McGee H, Zwisler AD, *et al*. Cardiac rehabilitation in Europe: results from the European Cardiac Rehabilitation Inventory Survey. *Eur J Cardiovasc Prev Rehabil* 2010: 17:410–18.

Cossette S, Frasure-Smith N, Lesperance F. Clinical implications of a reduction in psychological distress on cardiac prognosis in patients participating in a psychosocial intervention program. *Psychosom Med* 2001; 63(2):257–66.

Martin BJ, Hauer T, Arena R, *et al*. Cardiac rehabilitation attendance and outcomes in coronary artery disease patients. *Circulation* 2012; 126:677–87.

Piepoli M, Corra U, Benzer W, *et al*. Secondary prevention through cardiac rehabilitation: from knowledge to implementation. A position paper from the Cardiac Rehabilitation Section of the European Association of Cardiovascular Prevention and Rehabilitation. *Eur J Cardiovasc Prev Rehabil* 2010; 17:1–17.

Piepoli MF, Corrà U, Adamopoulos S, *et al*. Secondary prevention in the clinical management of patients with cardiovascular diseases. Core components, standards and outcome measures for referral and delivery: a policy statement from the cardiac rehabilitation section of the European Association for Cardiovascular Prevention & Rehabilitation. Endorsed by the Committee for Practice Guidelines of the European Society of Cardiology. *Eur J Prev Cardiol*. 2014; 21(6):664–81.

Scott IA. Determinants of quality of in-hospital care for patients with acute coronary syndromes. *Dis Manag Health Outcomes* 2003; 11:801–16.

Taylor R, Brown A, Ebrahim S, *et al*. Exercise-based rehabilitation for patients with coronary heart disease: systematic review and meta-analysis of randomized controlled trials. *Am J Med* 2004; 116:682–92.

Chapter 21

Examples of initiatives in different care settings: community

Key messages

- Prevention and rehabilitation programmes set up in the heart of the community have a greater chance of reaching vulnerable and deprived groups where prevalence of CVD and CVD risk factors is high.
- Setting up programmes in non-medical settings requires careful consideration to be given to data protection, accident and emergency policy, and infection control.
- A clear referral pathway is essential together with engagement of all referral sources.

Summary

- This chapter identifies the steps to take in setting up and implementing a preventive cardiology programme in the community.

Introduction

To successfully recruit and manage priority groups for CVD prevention, programmes should be delivered in a setting that is easily accessible to the target population. This approach offers a great opportunity to reach vulnerable and deprived groups where the prevalence of CVD is known to be high.

The MyAction programme is an example of a community-based model of CVD prevention which integrates the care of all those at high CVD risk (heart score >5%, vascular disease, heart disease, TIA, and type-2 diabetes), together with their families in one convenient community setting. This model of prevention evolved from the EUROACTION study[1] which demonstrated that a nurse-managed, multidisciplinary, family-based programme could achieve healthier lifestyle changes and better risk factor control than usual care at 1 year.

This chapter draws on the experience of setting up a MyAction programme in the West of Ireland by Croí (http://www.croi.ie), a registered Irish heart and stroke charity in collaboration with Imperial College London. Established in 2009, this unique, evidence-based service model is effectively implementing best-practice in achieving CVD prevention guidelines, and represents an efficient use of resources.[3]

Key steps to setting up a preventive cardiology programme in the community

In setting up a preventive cardiology initiative it is important to establish a programme management plan, which details key phases: needs assessment, planning, implementation, and evaluation.

Needs assessment

A 'needs assessment' provides evidence about a population on which to plan services and address health inequalities. It forms a central component of grant and funding applications. It should include:

- a profile of the target patient population, examining the prevalence and burden of disease
- identification of the potential gaps in current services and how the proposed programme meets the identified needs
- the potential for cost savings and restructuring of existing hospital prevention programmes to develop a community-based model
- the evidence base for the proposed intervention, for example, the MyAction programme is based on the principles and protocols of the EUROACTION cluster RCT.[1]

Planning

- From the outset, engage the key stakeholders, which may include hospital departments (cardiology, vascular surgery, stroke, and endocrinology), general practice (GPs and practice nurses), public health consultants, primary care services, health commissioners, and representatives from relevant community groups.
- Develop a business case to help secure funding; see Box 21.1 for a description of a business case.
- Develop a programme implementation plan outlining budget, timescales, and expected outcomes.

Box 21.1 What is a business case?

A business case provides the reasoning for initiating a programme and is often required as part of a funding application. A business case should outline the following:

- Aim and objectives of the programme
- The rationale or programme justification
- Description of the proposed programme
- Required resources/budget
- Contribute to national and local targets for CVD prevention
- Contribute to reducing health inequalities
- Clinical governance and service quality
- Key outcome measures.

Box 21.2 Choosing a community venue—important considerations

Chose an appropriate venue in a location that is accessible to the population being targeted, for example, if you are targeting patients from lower socioeconomic groups, consider a venue in a known deprived area. A suitable venue could be a community centre, leisure centre, or an unused office space that could be adapted accordingly.

The following is a checklist to consider when choosing a venue:

- Does the venue have adequate space to accommodate the physical programme requirements and the volume of patients to be targeted? Physical requirements will include a private one-to-one consultation space and an area where patients can exercise safely.

- Is the venue easily accessible via public transport links (e.g. bus stop and/or train station) and is there adequate parking available?

- Do the opening and closing hours of the venue facilitate the working hours of the programme?

- Is there adequate heat, air conditioning, and ventilation?

- Is there a lift available if the identified space is above the ground floor?

- What insurance (public liability) arrangements are in place and can additional cover be obtained if necessary?

- Can the venue support the programme IT technical requirements, such as accessing patient blood results?

- Does the facility have the required health and safety and fire regulations in place?

- Identify a suitable community venue to base the programme; see Box 21.2.

- Recruit a highly motivated, nurse-led, multidisciplinary team (physiotherapist/ exercise specialist, dietitian, nurse specialist, and psychologist if possible) with the support of a local cardiologist or physician with an interest in preventive cardiology. The team should also include administrative and programme management support.

- Using evidence-based prevention guidelines,[2] establish the programme protocol identifying outcomes and key performance indicators.

- In collaboration with key stakeholders, identify the key high-risk patient groups to be targeted and the principal referral sources (see Fig. 21.1 for an example).

- Develop a standardized and efficient referral pathway which highlights the inclusion criteria for the programme (see Fig. 21.2 for an example).

- This could be made available on a quick reference desktop card which displays the European HeartScore risk estimation tool.

- Adopt a multiple of approaches to promote recruitment to the programme, targeting both the referral source and the patient population directly (see Box 21.3).

Since the community is a non-medical setting, careful consideration needs to be given to developing the following policies and procedures:

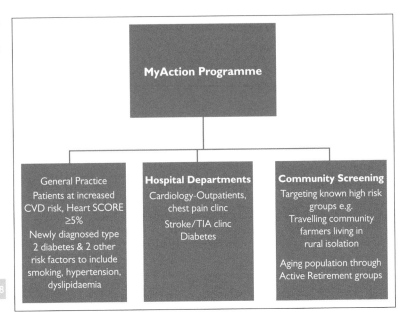

Figure 21.1 An example of the referral source for the MyAction programme.

Box 21.3 Recruitment to the programme—tips for success

- Develop a strong communication link with referral sources. This will involve regular meetings and working with referral sources in identifying high-risk patients in their practice/clinic.
- Promote and market the programme to the target population using social media, radio, press, public meetings, and other communication channels.
- Ensure all programme promotional materials are written in a language that is user friendly, are easy to interpret, and avoid the use of medical terminology. The benefits of attending the programme should be clearly identified and explicitly stated.
- Using specific pre-screening criteria, offer opportunistic screening/health checks in local community settings (e.g. supermarkets, community centres, and farmers' markets). This can be an effective way of reaching those most at risk as it removes the barrier of having to attend the GP/Hospital.
- Work in collaboration with leaders and key representatives from known high-risk, lower socioeconomic groups, inviting them to meet the multidisciplinary team, view the programme in action, and offer input to the patient recruitment strategy.

Step 1

Assess if the patient meets the inclusion criteria for the programme:

At high-risk for cardiovascular disease (CVD) according to Heart SCORE ≥5% (ESC Guidelines on CVD prevention 2012)

OR

Newly diagnosed type 2 diabetes and two other risk factors to include smoking, hypertension or dyslipidemia

Step 2

Inform patient about the MyAction programme (give information leaflet)
• Encourage patient to bring a supouse/partner or family member living in the same household to the programme
• Ask patient to contact MyAction to make an appointment within 1 week
• Complete the referral form and Email/Fax or Post the form to the MyAction Centre

Step 3

MyAction agrees an appointment time with the patient and a letter confirmin the appointment is sent to patient with a pre-assessment pack

Step 4

You will receive a letter of confirmation once the patient joins the programme

Step 5

Throughout the programme you will:
• Be updated on your patient's progress and clinical status
• Be informed if your patient is prescribed any cardioprotective medications or has medications adjusted while on the programme

Figure 21.2 Example of the referral pathway for use in general practice.

- Data protection—manage, store, and protect patient data in accordance with data protection guidelines; this may be done on site or in a central location.
- Accident and emergency protocol—ensure all staff are trained in cardiopulmonary resuscitation and the use of an automated external defibrillator which should be available on site.
- Infection control—outline procedures for phlebotomy and transport of blood samples to the local laboratory for analysis.

Implementation

- Adopt a flexible approach to delivery, offering a variety of programme and appointment times (e.g. evening and weekend).
- Ensure programme is being delivered to a high quality and standard, that is, it is protocol driven, evidence based, guideline orientated, and has appropriate clinical governance in place.
- Conduct regular staff training and performance reviews.
- Invite family members to participate in the programme.
- To help patients sustain lifestyle changes in the long term, work with local community groups and organizations in identifying suitable exit route opportunities such as walking groups, healthy cooking classes, smoking cessation groups, and so on.

Evaluation

- Conduct regular programme audits and monitoring of outcomes to ensure the programme is being delivered to the established protocol and guidelines.
- Ensure programme outcomes are being disseminated to key stakeholders and the appropriate funding bodies.
- To ensure the programme is meeting patient needs, it is important to obtain regular patient feedback.

Overcoming barriers to implementation

Identified barriers to implementation may include the following:

An inadequate project management plan

Implement practical project management tools to facilitate effective programme implementation, ensuring timescales and targets are met.

Low referral rates to programme

May be due to concern over referring to a non-conventional medical setting such as the community, lack of familiarity with prevention guidelines, and additional time involved in making the referral to the programme.

- Communicate with referral sources that appropriate programme governance and clinical support is in place.
- Adopt an integrated approach to care linking with both hospital and general practice. Ongoing liaising and communication with referral sources is essential.

For example, keeping the GP and practice nurse updated in relation to progress of patient and changes in prescribing regimen will foster a positive working relationship.

- As part of the programme set up, visit the referral source (hospital, primary care centre). This visit could be used as an opportunity to educate and update on prevention guidelines, describe the referral pathway, and assist in identifying patients at risk in the practice.
- Develop a user-friendly information pack for the referral source; this should contain a description of the programme, the referral criteria and pathway, patient information leaflets, and posters to be displayed in practice/clinic.
- Invite the referral sources to come and view the setting in which the programme is being delivered and to meet the multidisciplinary team.
- Offer continuing medical education accredited educational workshops/meetings surrounding prevention guidelines.
- Ensure the referral pathway is easy to interpret and where possible link with existing IT infrastructure to ensure efficient referral.

Inadequate support from key stakeholders

This will impact on the overall success of the programme:

- Appoint a medical director to the programme—ideally a local cardiologist or GP/physician with an interest in preventive cardiology.
- Establish a steering group for the programme, with defined goals and objectives from the early stage of programme planning.
- Report regularly to the steering group and referral sources on the progress of the programme.

Ethnicity and cultural beliefs

- Ensure programme materials are available in a range of languages that meet the requirements of the referral population.
- Consider the literacy levels of the target population.
- Consider use of interpreters where appropriate.

References

1. Wood D, Kotseva K, Connolly S, et al. Nurse-coordinated multidisciplinary, family-based cardiovascular disease prevention programme (EUROACTION) for patients with coronary heart disease and asymptomatic individuals at high risk of cardiovascular disease: a paired, cluster-randomised controlled trial. Lancet 2008; 371(9629):1999–2012.

2. Perk J, De Backer G, Gohlke H, et al. European Guidelines on cardiovascular disease prevention in clinical practice (version 2012). The Fifth Joint Task Force of the European Society of Cardiology and Other Societies on Cardiovascular Disease Prevention in Clinical Practice (constituted by representatives of nine societies and by invited experts). Eur Heart J 2012; 33:1635–701.

3. Gibson I, Flaherty G, Cormican S, et al. Translating guidelines to practice: findings from a multidisciplinary preventive cardiology programme in the west of Ireland. European Journal of Preventive Cardiology 2014; 21(3):366–376.

Chapter 22

Ensuring quality of interventions

Key messages

- Healthcare should be provided in an effective, timely, safe, and patient-oriented way.
- Healthcare providers are responsible for monitoring the quality of their services and ensuring they conform to a high standard.
- Outcomes should be developed and measured according to evidence summarized in guidelines to demonstrate quality.
- Preventive initiatives should be set up to include core components which take account of structure, process, and outcomes.
- Contribution of your service to clinical audit at national and regional level facilitates an awareness of how well your service performs compared to others.

Summary

- This chapter defines the concept of quality assurance and improvement and describes existing initiatives that measure quality of care.

Introducing the concept of quality and quality improvement

Healthcare should be provided in an *effective, timely, safe*, and *patient-oriented* way (see Box 22.1). Healthcare providers should be aware of the need for improvements in the quality of their services and should formally monitor maintenance of quality standards and improvements.

What are the indicators of quality, and how can we measure it and monitor its improvement?

For the purposes of measuring quality improvement, healthcare is classified as follows (see Fig. 22.1):

- Structure
- Process
- Outcome.

- *Effective*—achieving the desired outcomes.
- *Timely*—available to patients and their families when they need them: no waiting lists!
- *Safe*—for example, dependent on appropriate risk stratification, safe transport to and from the venue available.
- *Patient oriented*—for example, delivered on days and at times when it is convenient for patients and families to attend, tailored to their needs.

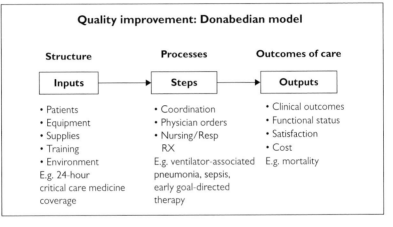

Quality improvement: Donabedian model

Structure	Processes	Outcomes of care
Inputs	**Steps**	**Outputs**
• Patients	• Coordination	• Clinical outcomes
• Equipment	• Physician orders	• Functional status
• Supplies	• Nursing/Resp	• Satisfaction
• Training	RX	• Cost
• Environment	E.g. ventilator-associated	E.g. mortality
E.g. 24-hour	pneumonia, sepsis,	
critical care medicine	early goal-directed	
coverage	therapy	

Figure 22.1 Structure, process, outcome.
http://openi.nlm.nih.gov/detailedresult.php?img=2738304_IJCCM-12–67-g001&req=4

Using these classifications helps to focus on the essential components of care and to ensure that all aspects are covered.

Standards and outcome measures

Measuring quality of care depends on there being 'a level of attainment' or *standard* and an expected health state, which results from a healthcare intervention, or *outcome measure*. See Box 22.2 for an example.

Evidence-based clinical guidelines

Guidelines provide standards and outcome measures based on evidence. The ESC hosts a programme of clinical guidelines development, which brings specialist and professional groups together to review and summarize the evidence base for interventions in cardiovascular care.

- *Standard*: to achieve preventive care in accordance with that defined in the European guidelines on prevention of CVD in clinical practice
- *Outcome measures*: for example, BP control of <140 mmHg SBP/90 mmHg DBP in all patients with established CVD or those at high cardiovascular risk and <140 mmHg SBP/85 mmHg DBP in patients with diabetes.

Quality can thus be measured against standards, which are set according to best evidence balanced with cost, which depends on the health economy of a country.

The ESC European Association for Cardiovascular Prevention and Rehabilitation hosts the Joint European Society's Taskforce (see Fig. 22.2) which is responsible for developing and updating the clinical guidelines on prevention of CVD (see Fig. 22.3).

This guideline supports the development of national guidelines in European countries and guides the development of appropriate interventions to address preventive care.

Core components

The set-up, delivery, and evaluation of preventive cardiology programmes are also aided by the development of *core components* that are essential and indispensable to ensuring the quality of an intervention.

FIFTH JOINT EUROPEAN SOCIETIES' TASK FORCE ON CARDIOVASCULAR DISEASE PREVENTION IN CLINICAL PRACTICE

- European Society of Cardiology (ESC)
- European Atherosclerosis Society (EAS)
- International Society of Behavioural Medicine (ISBM)
- European Stroke Organisation (ESO)
- European Society of Hypertension (ESH)
- European Association for the Study of Diabetes (EASD)
- European Society of General Practice/Family Medicine (ESGP/FM/WONCA)
- International Diabetes Federation Europe (IDF-Europe)
- European Heart Network (EHN)

Figure 22.2 The Joint European Societies Prevention Taskforce.

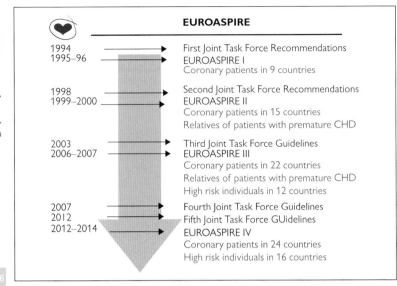

Figure 22.3 Timeline for guideline development and its audit.
Republished with permission of the ESC.

Core components should include *structure-based measures* offering guidance on types of infrastructure, equipment, personnel and training; and *process-based measures* offering guidance on the processes to include (see Box 22.3).

Outcome based measures would specify clinical outcomes based on national or regional evidence-based guidelines.

Audit: principles and examples

What is audit?

The *Oxford English Dictionary* defines 'audit' as a systematic review or assessment of something. In relation to clinical care, 'clinical audit' has been defined as: 'a quality

Box 22.3 Process-based measures for cardiovascular prevention and rehabilitation

- Referral pathways which promote recruitment of all eligible patients
- Individualized assessment of lifestyle and risk factors
- Individualized interventions to modify lifestyle and risk factors
- Progress monitoring plan
- Risk stratification for exercise
- Symptom monitoring
- Outcome monitoring and evaluation of programme effectiveness.

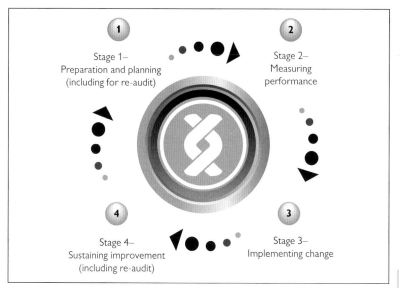

Figure 22.4 Audit cycle.

improvement process that seeks to improve patient care and outcomes through systematic review of care and the implementation of change' (http://www.hqip.org.uk, endorsed by NICE).

It provides:

- an objective assessment of clinical outcomes
- information on the process of care and the extent to which daily clinical practice is being implemented according to standards (i.e. according to evidence-based guidelines).

How to conduct audit

Audit is the process whereby quality improvement is assessed against standards and outcome measures. Audit has been described as a cycle (see Fig. 22.4), which includes the measurement of performance against standards of care and integrates the implementation of changes to improve care. Audit facilitates the monitoring of sustained improvement and always includes re-audit.

Clinical audit conducted at local service level is important for informing service delivery needs. In addition, it can contribute to audit at national or regional level (e.g. in a 'registry' or 'national audit') which allows comparison between centres providing services, whilst at the same time providing a national or regional picture of service provision. Research studies in the form of surveys can also inform quality improvement in the same way as clinical audit as long as they are representative of the area and population under study and have sufficient statistical power (see Box 22.4).

- Service level—for example, your own practice, cardiovascular prevention, and rehabilitation programme.
- National or regional level—for example, all cardiovascular prevention and rehabilitation programmes in one country, national registry.
- Research level—surveys.

- Clinical audit can also measure change over time during the course of an intervention and also to what extent these changes are sustained in the longer term.
- Picking up change depends on the use of outcome measures which are sensitive to small changes.
- Box 22.5 shows an example of outcome measures to include for a cardiovascular prevention and rehabilitation programme.
- Defined outcome measures and standards should be accompanied by treatment protocols and algorithms which guide professionals in achieving targets (see Fig. 13.3 in Chapter 13 for an example of a protocol relating to BP management).

- Self-reported smoking status validated with breath carbon monoxide ≤6 ppm.
- Adherence to the Mediterranean diet as measured by a score (see 'Mediterranean diet score' and Table 11.1 in Chapter 11).
- Achieving physical activity guideline of 30 minutes or more of moderate intensity physical activity on at least 5 days per week.
- Weight loss of at least 5% or more in individuals who are overweight (BMI 25–30 kg/m^2) or obese (BMI ≥30 kg/m^2).
- Ideal waist circumference <88 cm in women and <102 cm in men.
- SBP <140 mmHg and DBP <90 mmHg in all patients with established CVD or those at high cardiovascular risk and SBP <140 mmHg and DBP <85 mmHg in patients with diabetes.
- LDL-C <1.8 mmol/L (<70 mg/dL) in patients at very high cardiovascular risk, and <2.5 mmol/L (<100 mg/dL) in patients at high cardiovascular risk.
- HbA1c <7% (<53 mmol/mol) in patients with diabetes.
- Hospital Anxiety and Depression Scale (HADS) score.
- Global Mood Scale score.
- EQ-5D and EQ-VAS scores (EuroQol).
- Illness perception questionnaire—IPQ-R.
- Risk perception.

Some examples of audit

EUROASPIRE

- The ESC set up the Euro Heart Survey Programme in 1999, now the EurObservational Research Programme. The EUROASPIRE cross-sectional surveys of preventive cardiovascular care in coronary and high CVD risk patients were started in 1995 in order to evaluate guideline implementation after the publication of the first prevention guidelines in 1994. Euroaspire was a precursor to this ESC registry and subsequently became a part of it.

- These surveys are an example of how research can be used to assess and monitor quality improvement in care. They are conducted in regions within European countries and they recruit consecutively identified coronary patients from tertiary centres and district general hospitals and patients at high cardiovascular risk from general practices.

- Also included in the second and third surveys were first-degree relatives of patients with premature coronary disease, and the third and fourth surveys have included patients at high cardiovascular risk identified in general practice. The main outcome measures of these surveys are proportions of patients achieving lifestyle, risk factor, and therapeutic targets defined in the guidelines with data collection being based on a review of patients' medical notes at least 6 months after their acute event or commencement of risk factor modifying treatment, and also on an interview and examination. The surveys have been periodically repeated following publication of guideline updates (see Fig. 22.3).

- Central training for all investigators and field workers ensures the use of standardized methods for data collection using standardized equipment, whilst blood analyses are carried out in a central laboratory. Data are entered onto a web database and all data management is carried out from the ESC headquarters in Nice. All statistical analyses are conducted in Ghent in Belgium.

- This audit of preventive cardiology care has shown not only that care can be suboptimal, but has also revealed substantial variations in availability and provision of cardiovascular and prevention services, and in prescribing of cardioprotective medications. Comparison between surveys shows interesting trends of increasing obesity and prevalence of diabetes, reflecting those in the general population.

SURF

The SURF (SUrvey of Risk Factors) programme was set up in 2009 as a complement to the more expensive and time-consuming EUROASPIRE surveys as a simple, quick, and economical audit of preventive care that could be widely applied and represent practice throughout Europe and beyond (see Fig. 22.5).

The advantages of this method are as follows:

- The audit of an individual's care uses a one-page audit form (easily reproduced in an electronic format) (see Tables 22.1 and 22.2) and can be conducted within 90 seconds at a routine clinic attendance.

- This brevity may minimize selection and participation bias because there is no requirement to make a special time-consuming visit.

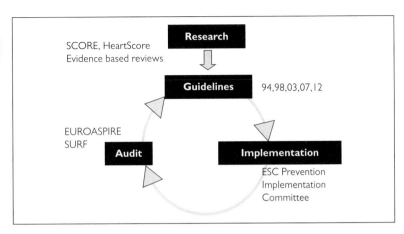

Figure 22.5 e-Surf.
Reproduced with permission from http://www.hqip.org.uk

- It would allow annual or bi-annual repeat surveys to audit secular changes in risk factor control.
- At each centre, starting from a defined date, risk factor information is collected on 10 to 50+ consecutive subjects attending the OPD with established CHD.

A SURF pilot has been conducted in three European and four Asian countries. The first phase of the project has seen the inclusion of more countries from both Europe and Asia with more to be included in the future. SURF is currently limited to an audit of secondary prevention although plans are in place to extend to primary prevention, and stroke.

The UK National Audit of Cardiac Rehabilitation

The National Audit of Cardiac Rehabilitation (NACR) provides an example of an audit conducted at national level under the auspices of the British Association for Cardiovascular Prevention and Rehabilitation (BACPR) and the British Heart Foundation. All cardiac rehabilitation programmes in the United Kingdom are encouraged to submit their data to this national database in an attempt to create a national picture of service provision.

In addition, it allows comparison across programmes because the same validated measures of dietary adherence, physical activity levels, and health-related quality of life are used.

Patient data are collected at programme entry, after completion of the programme and at 1 year. A questionnaire is also sent out to all programmes annually to collect data on staffing and the number of patients in each diagnostic category recruited to the programmes.

The audit is hosted by the University of York. The minimum dataset includes the following:

- *Demographic*—gender, date of birth, postcode, and ethnic status (national census method)

Table 22.1 e-Surf audit form 1

Demographics				
Initials:		Date of birth:		Hospital Name:
Gender:	☐ Male	☐ Female		MRN:
CHD Category:	☐ CABG	☐ PCI	☐ Acute coronary syndrome	☐ Stable AP	Date of examin:
Was the patient admitted to hospital in the last year with for a CHD related reson? ☐ Yes ☐ no				☐ Public patient ☐ Private patient
Risk factory history				**Most recent risk factory measurements**
Smoking history	☐ current smoker ☐ Ex smoker ☐ Never smoked			Systolic BP mmHG
				Diastolic BP mmHg
				Heart rate bpm
Physical activity	☐ Less than below ☐ Moderate (walking or equivalent) 30 mins 3 to 5 times per week ☐ More than this			Waist circumference cm
				Height m
				Weight kg
At what age did the patient complete full time education?	—— Years			Fasting bloods with in 1 year? ☐ Yes ☐ No
				If yes, date of fasting bloods:

(continued)

Table 22.1 Continued

Demographics				
Known history of (Patient was told of diagnosis previously)	Yes	No		
	☐	☐	Hepertension	
	☐	☐	Dyslipidaemia	
	☐	☐	Diabetes type 2	
	☐	☐	Diabetes type 1	
			Fasting total chol	mmol/l
			Fasging LDL chol	mmol/l
			Fasting HDL chol	mmol/l
			Fasting triglycerides	mmol/l
			Fasting glucose	mmol/l
Did the patient ever participate in cardiac rehab?	☐ Yes, fully or in part		HbA1C (if diabetic)	%
	☐ No			

Medications		
☐ Any anti-platelet	☐ Any ACE inhibitor	☐ Any nitrate
☐ Any statin	☐ Any Ca antagonist	☐ Any diuretic	☐ Any insulin
☐ Any other lipid lowering agent	☐ Any other anti-hypertensive	☐ Any ARB	☐ Any oral hypoglycaemic agent

Table 22.2 e-Surf audit form 2

Demographics

Initials:		Hospitals:	
Date of birth:		MRN:	
Gender:	☐ Male ☐ Female	Date of examination:	
Study Eligibility & CHD Category:	• Patient is eligible for study if they have objectively confirmed CHD with or without admission to hospital • PCI includes elective or emergency. • Acute coronary syndrome indicates candiac chestpain at rest with objective evidence of acute ischaemia or infarction • Stable AP = Clinical angina with objective confirmation from a clearly positive exercise ECG or ischaemia on perfusion imaging, or a coronary angiogram showing a narrowing of 70% or more in at least one coronary artery • Mark all diagnoses that apply.		

	Risk factory history	Most recent risk factory measurements	
Smoking history	Considered ex smoker if quit smoking more than 6 month ago Considered a smoker if any smoking now or in the last six month	Systolic BP Diastolic BP Heart rate	Complete with information from day of out patient visit – can be measured by nurse
Physical activity	Mark on answer only Other activities equivalent to walking include: golf, swimmin, etc.	Waist circumference Height Weight	

(continued)

Table 22.2 Continued

Demographics			
At what age did the patient complete full time education?	Enter age in years		
Known history of (Patient was told of diagnosis previously)	Mark "Yes" if the patient was previously told that they had this risk factor self reported information only is requierd	Fasting bloods with in 1 year?	☐ Yes ☐ No
		Date of fasting bloods (Most recent within 1 year)	
		Fasting total chol Fasting LDL chol Fasting HDL chol Fasting triglycerides Fasting glucose	Complete with most recent fasting bloods if taken within 1 year – *otherwise leave blank*
Did the patient ever partici-pate in cardiac rehab?	Self report of attendance	HbA1C (if diabetic)	
Medications			
Mark the drug class if the patient is taking it currently. Do not write in drug name or does. Do not write in drugs which the patient is taking which are not listed.			

- *Clinical*—BP, weight, height, cholesterol, medication, initiating event (reason for rehabilitation), previous cardiac events, and co-morbidities
- *Behavioural*—smoking status, activity level, economic activity measures from National Census, and physical fitness
- *Health-related quality of life*—as scored via the Dartmouth COOP questionnaire
- *Mental health*—anxiety and depression as scored via the HADS
- *Wait time*—date of initiating event, date referred to cardiac rehabilitation, date invited to join, date started rehabilitation programme, and date finished

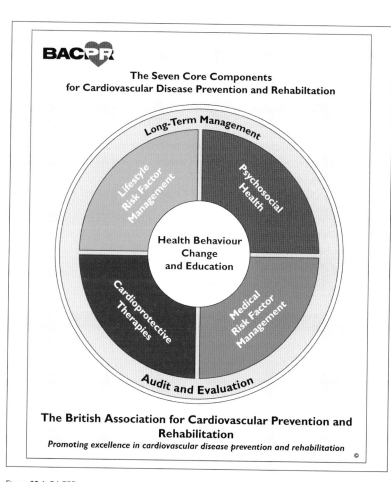

Figure 22.6 BACPR core components.
Republished with permission from BACPR.

- *Uptake*—agreed to take part (yes, no) and reason for refusal/being unable to attend
- *Drop-out rates*—reason for not completing cardiac rehabilitation, if known.

Examples of core components

Core components for cardiovascular prevention and rehabilitation have been developed on a European level with the EACPR Policy Statement.[1] In the United Kingdom, the BACPR have also developed minimum standards and core components (see Fig. 22.6 and Box 22.6).

Developing a dataset to record and monitor your process and outcome data

A dataset should include all the necessary variables, which will facilitate recording and monitoring to demonstrate adherence to core components and treatment protocols.

For example, Table 22.3 shows an example from the European core components[1] proposed data collection tool for diet and nutrition counselling. This could be further enhanced by the addition of a validated tool to assess adherence to a Mediterranean diet, that is, the Mediterranean diet score (see 'Mediterranean diet score' and Table 11.1 in Chapter 11).

Data should be recorded at appropriate time points to demonstrate effectiveness of interventions to facilitate change and improvement in those participating:

- At the start and end of an initiative or intervention
- In the long term (e.g. 1-year follow-up)
- Continuously (e.g. to assess proportions of patients prescribed) and adhering to therapies in general practice.

Using a database

A secure database will facilitate:

- monitoring of recruitment
- tracking of changes in clinical measurements

Box 22.6 BACPR seven core components for cardiac rehabilitation

- Health behaviour change and education
- Lifestyle risk factor management:
  - Physical activity and exercise
  - Diet
  - Smoking cessation
- Psychosocial health
- Medical risk factor management
- Cardioprotective therapies
- Long-term management
- Audit and evaluation.

Table 22.3 Sample data collection tool for the performance and outcome measurements of each component during and after a cardiac rehabilitation programme (example of diet and nutrition counselling)

Diet/nutritional counselling	Wide variety of foods; low salt foods; Mediterranean diet	—Optimal control —Suboptimal control	Applies to all patients with CVD: Education completed: —Target food goals —Lifestyle modification	Complete only if suboptimal control on initial assessment: —Patient encouraged to contact healthcare provider about reassessment	Policy is in place to communicate with healthcare providers as needed

- data analysis
- automated generation of letters used to communicate with patients, GP, and so on
- recording of data in a consistent and standardized manner
- enabling use of internal validation measures to promote accuracy of the data collected
- avoiding problem with missing data.

What is your role as a healthcare professional?

- To ensure that your service is audited
- That you act on audit results to improve quality
- To be aware of regional and national audit data and how your service compares with others.

Pointers

- *Don't reinvent the wheel*—there are several existing validated tools available and examples of datasets
- *Coordinate efforts*—feed into existing registries and databases
- *Use standardized methods and tools.*

Key reading

BACPR. *2012 Standards and Core Components for Cardiovascular Disease Prevention and Rehabilitation.* [Online] http://www.bacpr.com/pages/page_box_contents.asp?pageID=791

Donabedian A. The quality of care. How can it be assessed? *JAMA* 1988; 260:1743–8.

European Society of Cardiology. For information on EUROASPIRE see http://http://www.escardio.org/

National Audit of Cardiac Rehabilitation (NACR). NACR reports can be found at http://www.cardiacrehabilitation.org.uk

Perk J, De Backer G, Gohlke H, *et al*. European Guidelines on cardiovascular disease prevention in clinical practice (version 2012). The Fifth Joint Task Force of the European Society of Cardiology and Other Societies on Cardiovascular Disease Prevention in Clinical Practice (constituted by representatives of nine societies and by invited experts). *Eur Heart J* 2012; 33:1635–701.

Reference

1. Piepoli MF, Corrà U, Adamopoulos S, *et al.* Secondary prevention in the clinical management of patients with cardiovascular diseases. Core components, standards and outcome measures for referral and delivery: a policy statement from the cardiac rehabilitation section of the European Association for Cardiovascular Prevention & Rehabilitation. Endorsed by the Committee for Practice Guidelines of the European Society of Cardiology. *Eur J Prev Cardiol* 2014; 21(6):664–81.

Index

219